CW00468676

From Chronic

to Freed

Healing the Mind to Heal the Body,

Healing the Body to Heal the Mind.

A Journey of Transformation from

Illness to Profound Wellness

Jill Dunsford

BSc, Grad Dip Phys, MCSP, ONC (Hons)

Disclaimer

The information in this book is not a substitute for and is not to be relied on for medical or healthcare advice. Please consult your medical practitioner before changing, stopping or starting any medical treatment or therapy. The information given in this book is an account of the author's own experiences and the author does not hold any liability arising directly or indirectly from the use or misuse of the information in this book.

Contents

Acknowledgments

I have not travelled this journey alone, and there are many people I want to thank for guiding me and helping me.

First, I would like to thank Jill White, who, at the Riding for the Disabled meeting, told me about spiritual healing and the Doctor Healer Network. This led me initially to Peter Saywood.

Then, thanks to the Doctor Healer Network, where I met Wendy Walling, my hypnotherapist.

Next on my thank list is my dear friend, Anne Grayson, who introduced me to "The Journey "and Brandon Bays. Around this time, I also learned of Sai Baba, who supported me from far away throughout my journey.

I would also like to thank organisations such as HeartMath, The Flow Genome Project, and Fundamental Wellbeing. All of these helped me to discover and live in flow states and find my authentic self.

I'm grateful to my editor from knliterary, Sarah Bossenbroek. Of course, you wouldn't be reading this if not for Sarah's expertise and I am also grateful to the team at Savvy Books in bringing this book to you.

I also thank Hay House Publishing for allowing me to quote from "Mind to Matter" by Dawson Church 2018 Hay House, Inc., Carlsbad, CA, and Sentient Publishing for granting permission to quote from Thorwald Dethlefsen and Ruediger Dahlke, The Healing Power of Illness: Understanding What Your Symptoms Are Telling You (Boulder, CO: Sentient Publications, 2016).

I would also like to thank everyone I met, including friends and family, who acted as mirrors and signposts on the way and finally, my husband. Having looked after my mother in her last years, I know it can be as hard to be in the role of carer as it is of the sufferer.

About the Author

The author, was working as a Chartered Physiotherapist in the NHS, when she fell ill with a viral infection from which she didn't recover. After six years of suffering and finding no help in orthodox medicine, she decided to take the responsibility of rehabilitation into her own hands and to look for help outside the western medical paradigm.

This is the story of her transformation from chronic fatigue to recovery.

Introduction

When I first became ill, back in 1984, myalgic encephalomyelitis, otherwise known as chronic fatigue syndrome, was almost unheard of—or at least, I hadn't heard of it before. So why has it become so much more prevalent now?

As I write this, many people around the world are experiencing long Covid, with some symptoms similar to ME/CFS. And it makes one wonder why our immune systems don't deal with these bugs properly these days. Why didn't you or I recover? What's going on?

In the beginning, I kept meeting people who would tell me I had to learn to live with it and that it's incurable. However, today my experience says otherwise.

This is my story of transformation, from illness and prior feelings of inadequacy and despair to happiness and a deep sense of well-being. Although I am not advocating any treatment or approach, this is a first-hand account of what I found worked for me.

If I can recover, so can you!

I had known for a long time that I wanted to write this book, but I didn't know how best to approach it; should I write an autobiography or just about therapies? Many years ago, after I had recovered, I had a dream in which I was writing a book about all the various gardening techniques I

1

used. When I woke up, I realised that I needed to substitute healing for gardening.

It's taken me many years to get around to writing it—one reason being that my approach to healing has been so unique. There was no model out there for me to work from. In the end, I decided to confine myself to what had worked for me, with personal examples. I was and still am my own lab rat.

People with ME/CFS find it hard to read for long periods, so I have tried to include as much information as possible while keeping it concise and interesting. I'll discuss why I think that people with ME/CFS find reading difficult in the chapters that follow.

I think healing for ME/CFS can only be done truly effectively by using a holistic approach. In fact, probably all patients with chronic diseases might be able to benefit from this approach. I understand that many ME/CFS sufferers may choose to read this in the order it's written or that they may prefer to jump around. For this reason, some of what I've written has been reiterated—so feel free to choose whether to skip over a repeated bit or use it as a refresher.

This back-and-forth method of flipping through this book is also a mirror for what may need to be done for recovery as well. Sometimes it may well feel like two steps backwards for every one forward, and, as I will explain later in the book, our symptoms can have many layers.

Since I first developed ME/CFS, there has been much more medical research on the disease, as it is now recognised as a physical disease, and there are more ideas and helpful approaches available for the patients to try. There was very little (bordering on none) when I first developed it. In hindsight and maybe rather curiously, I am extremely grateful for this fact. That there wasn't a magic pill has proved to be a disguised blessing.

Even with this new approach—that it's a physical disease—many people remain ill for years. According to ME Research, a UK-based organisation, some 17 million people worldwide have some degree of chronic fatigue. There's a wide range of symptoms, and the tests used by doctors mostly come back negative, which leads sufferers to ask the question, "What's wrong with me?"

When I first got ill, I was encouraged to learn to live with it, and a recent search for books on "ME/CFS" on the website of a well-known online bookseller indicates that this still seems to be the predominant approach.

But regardless of what anyone told me, I was not going to learn to live with it. I was going to get over it. In fact, even suggesting I learn to live with it felt like a slap in the face. I was in my mid-30s, and to spend the rest of my life like this was a thought that I was not ready to entertain. So I told myself - No way!

During my search for healing, I came across many people who didn't believe that recovery was possible, and I remember hearing a well-known personality declaring to an audience of hundreds that it was incurable. This statement angered me. I believe people in influential positions need to be very careful about what they say.

"Whether you think you can, or you think you can't—you're right." —Henry Ford

After six years of waiting and hoping for an orthodox cure, I woke up one morning and decided I would do something, anything, even if it killed me. I was no longer prepared to live this shadow of a life. So, I decided to take action and started looking for other ways to recover through complementary and alternative therapies.

If you have eliminated all other potential causes for your fatigue, such as toxic black mould in your home, dental amalgam toxicity or electromagnetic pollution, then you may want to take this approach.

I have written it for all of you who also choose not to "live with it." The path I share with you has taken me from illness and despair to happiness and well-being.

May you be happy

May you be well

May you be free from fear

May you be at peace

May you be full of loving-kindness

Loving-Kindness meditation

Chapter 1: Descent into Darkness

I date the onset of my illness at the time I had my first panic attack, but it had actually probably started a few weeks before. At first, I developed a rash down the outside of my left leg and a swollen lymph node in my groin. As I worked in close proximity to people, I went to see my doctor to find out if what I had was contagious, and he told me that I probably had shingles. The rash, which followed the path of a nerve, was very sensitive to touch, but as I felt well and was apparently unlikely to be infectious, I continued to work.

Looking back, I now realise that the onset may have even started before this. For several months, I had been having sudden visions about being involved in a car accident and breaking my thigh and interruptive thoughts such as "stop the world, I want to get off." In the end, I was stopped big-time by this disease, and it took a lot longer to recover from it than it would have from breaking my leg.

A few days later, I woke up feeling very unwell following a heavy night out with friends. And, having the mindset that self-abuse is not a reason to skip work, I went in.

My job entailed working in outlying clinics, to which we drove on a daily basis. While I was being driven by my colleague to the hospital where I was to work that day, I started to feel seriously unwell. I felt nauseous, faint and dizzy. I started sweating and had double vision to the point that I started wondering if I was dying. By the time I got to the clinic, my heart was racing, and it was then that I really thought I was dying. I was terrified by this stage and, after a short while, took myself to the emergency department.

The on-duty nurse took my pulse—140 beats per minute. The doctor came in, took a brief history, told me I was having a panic attack, turned around and walked out. I said to myself that I'm not the type to have panic attacks. Cool, calm and collected—that's me.

The day after the initial diagnosis of a panic attack, I woke up with an ache in my left arm. I still felt nauseous, anxious, tense and ill. Remembering my medical training, I wondered if I had heart issues. At times I found myself with tears pouring down my face, my heart skipping beats—even slight exertion caused my heart to race. My body felt as if there was a small electric motor running continuously, and I was very jumpy. Over the next few days, I found that when it was hot, I was cold, and when it was cold, I was hot. I had night sweats, and if I didn't get to bed by 6 pm, I couldn't get to sleep until about 3 am. My blood sugar balance was all over the place, and I could even feel faint and dizzy lying completely flat. I remained tense and anxious all the time.

So I decided to make an appointment to see my doctor again. He told me it takes a little longer to recover from such an illness now that I am older. I looked at him in astonishment. I was 34, not 94. He was, however, right. It did take some years.

I went and saw another doctor as I wasn't getting the help I believed I needed. He told me I did not have shingles but that I did have myocarditis. He assured me that I would be okay in six months and advised me not to overdo things. That came as a relief until six months later, when I was no better, and so I then arranged to see a cardiologist.

I overheard him ask my general practitioner if I was neurotic. He was told that no, I was not. After examining me and the results of my ECG (EKG), he told me that I never had myocarditis.

I lost weight, and at times I looked grey and gaunt. I was constantly feeling ill—sometimes more ill, sometimes less, but always and continuously ill. I felt as though I might drop dead any minute.

If I hadn't been so scared of dying and death, I might as well have committed suicide. I could do anything, absolutely anything, to escape from the nightmare that had become my life.

If I needed to eat, it was an urgent need to eat right then, not in five minutes—now. By necessity, I became totally controlling of others, anything to limit my symptoms. What a nightmare for them. I was bewildered, confused and lost.

There is this weird phenomenon in ME/CFS of "doing too much." There is a "line", and to cross it by even one step is to put you in bed for a day, a week, or longer. It was as if I had 100 pennies of energy to spend, and I could spend them all in one go and then do absolutely nothing for the rest of the day or spend them slowly over that day. But that was the extent of it. I could not get any extra energy by eating or resting unless it was a decent amount of sleep.

Sleep brought some respite, but only if I went to sleep by 6 pm. Any later, and I couldn't get to sleep for hours.

Even with all this going on, I continued to work. I was told it would take my mind off my problems. But every day, I would have face-to-face consultations with patients, and I couldn't focus. I would have to excuse myself, walk away and gather my thoughts to concentrate enough so that I could ignore all the weird feelings in my body and focus on them and their problems.

They would be telling me their issues, and inside I would be thinking, you ought to try what I'm feeling right now to know what a problem feels like!

I continued to struggle like this, as I felt that to resign was to admit failure, that I was broken, neurotic, and unfit. And on top of that, I really didn't even like my job. I had found that physiotherapy did not give me a sense of doing something useful or beneficial to people.

Fortunately, after three years, my husband was earning enough to support us both, so I finally resigned. Then I got worse. I was all over the place, both physically and emotionally.

I was told of a diagnostic physician in London, and I made an appointment to go and see him. He examined me and looked horrified at the state I was in. He made an immediate appointment with another cardiologist, who we walked over to see. That doctor, in turn, arranged for me to be admitted to a private hospital. Fortunately, we had medical insurance. I was told I was hyperventilating, and the treatment prescribed was sedation-induced sleep.

After a few days of medically-induced rest, I felt much better and was discharged home. But upon arriving home, I was no better. This same treatment was repeated several months later in an NHS hospital. It didn't work this time either.

It was assumed by this cardiologist and his occupational therapy assistant that it was my relationship with my husband that was the root of the problem, and I should leave him. It wasn't, and I didn't.

I abandoned the hospital-based approach, as it was expensive and wasn't working.

Looking back now, I do sympathise with the doctors I met. In a world of materialistic medicine, if there are no definitive tests, there are challenges to diagnosis. The only positive test result I had showed that I had had a viral infection. They were as much in the dark as I was.

Even terms like ME/CFS or fibromyalgia don't tell you anything that you don't already know!

You go to the doctor and tell him you're tired all the time, and if there is no obvious cause like anaemia, you get told you have chronic fatigue. But you already know that. You've just told him or her that in the description of your symptoms.

- Myalgia: pain in the muscles
- Encephalomyelitis: inflammation of the brain
- Chronic fatigue syndrome: you're tired, but no one knows why
- Fibromyalgia: your muscles hurt

All these diagnoses just describe your symptoms with fancy words, but they don't help you get better.

As I was getting no help, I became totally self-absorbed in my problems and needed to control as much of my life as I could, from the food I ate to the people I interacted with. People stopped asking me out, as I could never commit. I didn't know how I would feel from one minute to the next. It was a nightmare for my husband and family.

After six years of my life becoming more and more restricted and waiting for an orthodox treatment to help me, I woke up one morning and decided enough was enough. I was no longer willing to live this shadow of a life.

Then, things started to happen.

May you be well

Chapter 2: Discovery and Recovery

My recovery took the form of numerous discoveries. The first one—there wasn't a pill.

If there had been a pill for this disease, I would have taken it. I'm not masochistic enough to enjoy being ill, and I was only 34 when I became ill. There was too much life still left for me to live. Looking back, however, I am quietly pleased that there wasn't a pill or a drug. This disease has taught me so much that it has, in all truth, been a gift. It might sound surprising, but it is true.

Many years ago, someone told me I would be ultimately grateful for it and indeed, I am. It has taken me from resentment, anger and anxiety to a deep sense of well-being. I even remember telling someone recently that as a young adult, I majored in resentment, and now I am in love with life. Who couldn't be grateful for that?

To arrive at this conclusion took a paradigm shift. But I am leaping ahead.

After I had made my decision to do something about my situation, a friend who helped at our local (horse) Riding for the Disabled Group came and asked me if I would like to help. I looked at her in astonishment as I could hardly stand, let alone walk for an hour with a pony and vulnerable rider.

She told me that she didn't want me to do anything active. All she wanted me to do was to sit and just give some advice, if appropriate, as a physiotherapist. She thought that I might have some advice on how to support the young adults and children, such as how best it is for the helpers to help them mount the horses, etc.

I agreed to give it a try, and I went and sat on the mounting block for an hour, giving pointers when necessary. Then I drove home and went to bed for the rest of the day because in just doing that small bit, I was exhausted.

The next week, I went along again and sat on the box for an hour. Just before I went home, the woman taking the class came up to me and started chatting. She explained that she was a novice spiritual healer. This was completely outside my experience up until that point in my life. I don't think I'd even heard about spiritual healing or knew that you could be a student in it.

She went on to say that sometimes spiritual healing was beneficial for people when orthodox medicine didn't have the answers. She couldn't take me on as a client, as she was too busy, but she told me about a weekend workshop happening in a couple of weeks, so I signed up for it.

I thought attending could pose quite a challenge because just sitting for an hour on the mounting block at the Riding for the Disabled events was hard enough. But I considered that it would be a community of healers, so they would be patient, kind and considerate people, so why not?

I went along. One of the presenters was a retired medical doctor, now a spiritual healer. The fact that he had worked in orthodox medicine and was now talking about spiritual healing made me take notice. I felt reassured that there was merit in this approach when I entered this uncharted territory. Nothing to date had helped, and I found his presence reassuring, despite my caution and scepticism. Maybe spiritual healing wasn't as flaky as I had thought.

The two workshop presenters started off by talking about more than our physical bodies. They included our spirits and our minds as part of our anatomy—concepts that were new to me.

I had trained in western orthodox medicine, the "pill for every ill" approach, but I had noticed the power of the mind to change people's outcomes—for good or bad. This workshop was the beginning of my understanding of the power of the mind to affect our physiology.

I remembered a patient who had surgery that wasn't that extensive or high-tech, but it was enough to keep him in the hospital for a few days to recover. A doctor on his rounds to do a standard post-op check on him listened to his lungs. The doctor told the patient that he had a mild case of pneumonia. Basically, he was just telling him that he had a slight chest infection—a common post-op event.

To this man, pneumonia was a potentially fatal disease, and when he heard that word, that's nearly what happened to him. Within 24 hours, he had gone down with pneumonia in both lungs and instead of being discharged in a matter of days, it took us six weeks to get him back up and ready to go home.

When he came back in for more surgery, we all said, "Don't tell him he's got pneumonia!" We understood that in his mind, the story was that pneumonia is a killer. He had his surgery, and he was home within the week.

From this and many other encounters, I knew that the mind could affect the body. What I didn't know was how that came about or in what ways my mind might be affecting me for good or ill.

Our minds are made up of two parts: the conscious mind and the unconscious mind. The conscious mind is the one that makes us aware of what is happening at the moment. We use it to access memories and think about current problems, for starters. The unconscious mind holds our feelings and memories—everything that has ever happened to us. It is also responsible for maintaining our physiological functions, such as breathing and digestion. Many of our behaviours also become unconscious.

The unconscious mind can also be further divided into two parts: the sympathetic, or "flight, fright, freeze" mind; and the parasympathetic, or "relax, digest and heal" mind.

The size of these two brains is vastly different, akin to an iceberg—One-third is visible, and two-thirds are beneath the sea. This can cause problems because we may consciously want to change a behaviour, but somewhere, sometime before, this particular behaviour may have been advantageous. It may have saved our life or felt like it had.

Many people get the idea that they are "not good enough." It may have been the result of perfectionist parents or teachers encouraging us to work harder or maybe being the younger sibling of a brother or sister a few years older with more skills. It's hard to be "not good enough," and so often, we work extra hard to reach "enough," but it sometimes still feels in vain. The message stored in our unconscious will always be "not good enough" until we make it conscious, accept its existence and can then challenge the underlying belief. This thought alone is stressful and sets up life for all sorts of health problems.

We become ill at ease, dis-eased.

We also can suppress these feelings by numbing them. But the problem with numbing out pain is that we are unable to cherry-pick pain. And in trying to numb the pain, we end up also numbing out joy and happiness. Numbing one emotion leads to numbing all.

We can try and suppress these hidden messages, which are felt in the body as discomfort, maybe emptiness, despair or a sense of failure. We cope by becoming a workaholic, or eating, smoking, gambling or drinking—anything that numbs these feelings but can only be a temporary solution. On the other hand, becoming aware sets us free.

"Know thyself." – Delphic Oracle

Many diseases in western medicine are treated with drugs, which is just another way of numbing out without solving the problem. Most often, the symptoms are looked upon as the disease for which a medication is given, and the symptom alleviated or suppressed—but the underlying root cause remains unaddressed.

Things are slowly changing toward a more holistic approach, and it is becoming acknowledged that stress is one of the major contributors to disease.

But where does the underlying cause of ME/CFS reside? In mind? In body? Or both?

I believe that the hallmark symptom of low energy occurs because so much energy is being used to suppress our pain. We are using our energy to block our feelings and using energy to block our emotions which, as the term emotion

18

(energy (e) in motion) implies, should be felt and allowed to move.

I acknowledge that this idea may be unpopular, but I came to it from my own experience. Every time I allowed myself to fully feel the feelings, accept the emotions and release or integrate them, I had more energy. And this didn't just happen once, but every time.

So, if this is what is happening, I am using energy to suppress my feelings. How do I discover what I am suppressing? Where will I find the answers? At this time, I didn't know where or how to look, or even how to feel, so how could I liberate my blocked energy?

May you be free from pain

Chapter 3: Discovery: All My Answers Are Within Me

"All your answers are within you."

My first spiritual healer kept saying this to me. Personally, I couldn't and still can't understand why people get so upset that ME/CFS was considered as "all in the mind." If it was, I could do something about it; maybe I could change my mind. At the time, I believed that if it was in my body, it was beyond my ability to do something about it. Fortunately, I was wrong about that.

My understanding is that the separation of mind and body is a historical quirk. This idea that the body and mind are separate has given rise to the modern mechanistic approach to medicine. But aren't you more than a machine?

If you see and smell a delicious meal, you will salivate. If you see a frightening film, your heart will start to beat faster, your mouth may dry up, and your body prepares to defend itself even though you are simply watching a film from the comfort of your home. You are in absolutely no danger, but your body reacts as though it is. The inputs to your mind change the state of your body.

"The fact that the mind rules the body is, despite of its neglect by biology and medicine, the most fundamental fact

that we know about the process of life." – Dr Franz Alexander

In the wonderful book, *The Body Keeps the Score* by Dr Bessel van der Kolk, he explains how a person's mind can fail to register the threat from an event, but the body doesn't. The unconscious mind keeps signalling to the body with stress hormones. The body remains in a perpetual state of flight, fright or freezes until the person gets so run down that they become ill.

Either a major one-off event or a drip, drip of constant minor stresses can lead to a collapse, as outlined by Dr. Van der Kolk. For us with ME/CFS, it is probably the latter. Our bodies are still registering the threat, and as Dr Sue Morter would say, "The trauma is over, but you feel as if the bears are still in the room."

Over the course of my years of living with ME/CFS, I consulted a few clinical psychologists in an effort to untangle what was going on in my mind. I remember one who kept asking me, "How did that make you feel?" After about 30 minutes of this, I got really annoyed and almost snarled, "I *don't* fucking feel!"

But of course, I did.

If you don't allow yourself to feel emotions, you will feel symptoms. As it says in The Healing Power of Illness: Understanding What Your Symptoms Are Telling You by

Thorwald Dethlefsen and Rüdiger Dalkhe, "Our symptoms make us honest."

What we are denying and suppressing is there for all to see and know—*if* you understand the language of the body.

"All in the mind" does not mean anyone imagines anything. It's not a figment, a fanciful creation to avoid life, living or responsibility. It is not hypochondria. Frankly, I wasn't that imaginative to think up all the symptoms I had— and why would I?

I had waited six years for a cure, to be told what was causing my disease and what it would take to get over it. I had waited in vain.

The day I woke up and decided I would try anything and everything, even if it killed me, was the day I took responsibility for my life. I wasn't going to live the rest of my life in this nightmare, this twilight existence. Afraid of going out, of eating the wrong food, of doing the wrong thing—afraid of everything. It was like being in prison and sitting on the side-lines of life while I just kept getting older. What sort of existence was that? Grim.

I was ill, and there didn't seem to be a cure. It wasn't my fault, but the least I could do was to take responsibility in the hope that I, maybe, could cure myself.

Discovery: The Power of the Unconscious Mind

I already knew I had two minds: a conscious one and an unconscious one. What I hadn't realised was the power of the unconscious mind. That is why so many of us self-sabotage. For example, our conscious mind says, "I want to give up comfort eating," while our unconscious mind will tell us to eat in order not to feel the pain or the feelings that our comfort eating suppresses.

It may sound a bit masochistic, but if we can face, welcome, and accept that pain, it will pass, and the need to comfort eat will stop. Otherwise, what we resist will persist.

"If you bring forth what is within you, what you bring forth will save you. If you do not bring forth what is within you, what you do not bring forth will destroy you." – The Gospel of St. Thomas

If "all my answers are within me," how did they get there? How do I find them?

Let's take a look from the beginning: Babies do not even know that they are separate beings. They have no recognition of where they end up and where their parent or caregiver begins. At this stage, they are unaware that they are a separate body, a separate being. They learn this slowly by biting their fingers and toes, exploring objects, the edges of their cots, and so on.

According to an eminent psychiatrist, Dr Stanislav Grof, babies can and do take on board and internalise their caregivers' feelings—even starting in utero, though this hypothesis is not always recognised by other psychiatrists.

At this stage of their development, they can have absolutely no awareness that these feelings are not theirs, that these feelings belong to someone else, but if the mother is traumatised or the baby feels it is not wanted, issues can arise later in the life of the child.

Small children are also very literal: they do not know when something might be threatening their survival or not. This is why they need to be taken care of—they don't yet have the "filters" that are created by life's teachings.

I am about four years old, and I hear a noise downstairs. I creep out of bed to listen, and I hear my father shouting at my mother, who is crying. I am feeling alone, abandoned, and unsafe. I feel there is no one to look after me.

At this age, I did not have the knowledge that this was just a temporary blip in their relationship and that they would likely reconcile. At this age, I did not have a proper filter to understand the situation, which may have passed harmlessly through me if I had been a bit older. I remained deeply stuck, left with a feeling of being unsafe, which I couldn't tolerate, so I ignored it as much as possible. But it remained there, affecting my behaviour.

There are many types of wounds within us, and this is just one example. Even if this was just a one-off occasion with very little or even no harm done, there could be a continuous tension in the parental relationship, which can be a problem for the child. The child may even feel responsible for this rift. No wonder I became a peacemaker (I will go into the effects of adverse childhood experiences in a later chapter).

By careful exploration with the help of my first healer and others later, including my hypnotherapist and *The Journey* with Brandon Bays, I was able to find my own answers, my own resources, and my own healing.

One of these ways is to explore the physical ways of finding answers. If I can pause, breathe, and become aware, I can break this pattern.

My left arm is aching, my hand feels uncomfortable.

I ask myself, "What am I feeling? What is the sensation? What is the emotion?"

This feeling is familiar, I wait and pay close attention to the sensations, what do they remind me of? What do they feel like? I sense a reluctance, a tightening in my abdomen, tension in my chest, my whole body wants to move backwards. Apprehension, I am feeling apprehensive. I don't want to receive something, experience something, and hold something.

I notice I am holding my breath, so I breathe and take awareness into my hand and arm, I observe with interest and curiosity. I welcome the feelings; I try to accept them. There is fear here, I accept that too. I welcome it.

The ache moves up into my forearm, my upper arm is tensing. What is this reminding me of? When have I felt like this before? My jaw is clenched, I am aware of anger and rage.

I want to lash out but also feel the resistance to expressing my anger. I am afraid to express my anger. I am ashamed of being angry.

I breathe into this, too; my body shakes itself, and I start to smile. Some of the emotions have dissipated. There is still an ache.

I continue the process, going deeper.

I can feel resentment, what is triggering that? What is beneath it? There is shame, and suddenly I know when this incident happened.

I am eight or nine years old and being shouted at by a teacher in front of everyone in the dining hall at school. She is calling me deceitful and sly.

I ask myself, what resources did I need at the time? Courage, integrity, nobleness. Giving myself these, the incident becomes inconsequential, and my arms ache goes away.

I am left feeling compassion toward the teacher. That comes as a big surprise!

It really can release this quickly. I remember once waking up with such severe sciatica. I thought I was going to be sick with the pain. I was just able to welcome it and breathe, and suddenly, with a flash of insight, the pain went. It was so startling; I nearly couldn't believe it. (I can't remember now what this insight was. One of the characteristics of this type of processing is that once it has been integrated, it "disappears."

After all, the body is no longer afraid, no longer resists, so it doesn't need it).

The left-arm ache was one of the first symptoms I developed with ME/CFS, and at the time, I wondered whether I had heart trouble. I got myself fully checked (ECG etc.) to rule out any heart problems. And although I eventually looked largely outside orthodox medicine for answers, I knew that there was certainly a place for orthodox treatment, particularly in acute situations.

I hope to see the day when western medicine embraces more than just the physical signs and symptoms, the day when it starts to teach people how to use their minds to heal. When it becomes holistic. Change your mind, and you change your physiology. Change your physiology, and you change your health.

There are positive signs that these ideas are being accepted and adopted. There is the discipline of psychoneuroimmunology, which acknowledges how stress, a mental phenomenon, affects our body's immune system and how stress is a major contributing factor to many diseases.

"All experiences are preceded by mind, having mind as their master, created by mind." – Gautama Buddha Dhammapada

When something horrid occurs, what usually happens is that we just react. Of course, we will. We react faster than we can think, but as soon as you notice you've reacted, if you can pause and breathe, you will be able to transform your experience of life. You will be able to heal your life.

So, how to get what is held within our bodies and memories out safely and without re-traumatising ourselves? I started to learn more ways on how and where to find my answers. More ways to learn how to heal.

May you be at peace

Chapter 4: My Body Wants to Heal

"Bodies heal," I knew this from years of experience. When I cut myself, my skin healed. When I broke my wrists, the bones healed. When I had a cold or flu, I healed. So, why was this not the case when I got ME/CFS?

Our bodies want to heal. Since the body is where trauma gets stored, it will keep reminding us of our traumas until we can discover the tools that we need to heal them; thus, restoring the body. These reminders are our symptoms. Unfortunately, most of us have not realised the connection between what we are feeling *now* and what happened *then*.

Maybe the question is not "what's wrong with you?" but "what happened to you?"

After all, the first question is simply asking for a list of your symptoms. While the second is an investigation to find the potential cause of your symptoms. It addresses you, the person who is in pain and not just as some kind of a machine that's malfunctioning.

To heal is to be made whole. To remember is to realise all that we are. To remember is literally to reintegrate those parts of us that we have abandoned, separated off, and repressed from our awareness. To re-member, as disease is dis-ease.

Awareness is key. We need to integrate the traumas that caused us to cut off the feelings and emotions we were unable to cope with at the time. To accept and own those parts of us –whether they are emotional, mental, or physical that we were told or we tell ourselves are unacceptable.

As children, stuff happened. Things that we couldn't handle, and as a result, a part of us is stuck at the age when that particular event occurred. It needs to be helped to grow up, and one way is to give your younger self the resources that you lacked at the time. If you were overwhelmed by fear, then give yourself the resource of courage and re-experience that incidence with this courage and see how it changes its effect on you.; knowing you had that courage can change everything. And of course, you can add any other resource that you might have needed at the time.

This changes how you experience your life; you cease to be afraid of the feelings or the experiences that you couldn't handle, they become integrated, that part grows up, and the symptoms disappear.

"When people change energetically, matter follows right along." – Dawson Church, Mind to Matter *2018*

Hay House, Inc., Carlsbad, CA

To change our minds and alter our belief systems, obviously, we must know what's in it. Meditation and mindfulness are very useful tools, and so is understanding the language of the body. What are your symptoms telling you?

At one time, when I was in a group of people (in a workshop, for example), and we had to introduce ourselves to the other group members, my heart would start to race, my mouth would dry up, and anxiety would arise. Why? All I was doing was saying my name and where I came from. Part of my recovery was discovering this memory:

I am about nine years old, and it is the first week of a new term at a school. I have only been here for one semester. I have been given an order mark which is a black mark on my record.

In my eyes, I had simply been protecting a friend, but the teacher didn't like my behaviour, hence the order mark. The day following this, there is a "house" meeting (British schools were often divided into houses for team competitions). I am made to stand up in front of 50 girls and confess my "crime" of being "shameful and deceitful,"— which is what the teacher called me.

From this day on, standing up and being conspicuous in a group of peers triggered my anxiety, causing a raised pulse and dry mouth. It also caused me to avoid criticism or any situations that might cause me shame, so anything that drew attention to me was challenging.

I know this happened. However, what I didn't know was that whenever my unconscious mind perceived a similar situation, even years later, as in this workshop example of just giving my name, all these symptoms would be triggered. In the workshop, I just felt very uncomfortable and confused. My unconscious mind saw the workshop situation as a threat. I could be pilloried, shamed, or potentially ostracised, so my body went into fight or flee mode (having found this and integrated it, I am now perfectly happy speaking in groups and teaching them).

So, you can see, it's not your fault, you were too young, too overwhelmed. There is no blame, just compassion—and responsibility—a responsibility to take back our power, which we have left behind attached to these traumas.

The unfortunate modern fixation on blaming everyone else is a mindset that turns us into victims. In this case, it's not your fault, and it's no one else's either. It's an unfortunate quirk that when bad things happen, we make decisions about them and set up belief systems. We do this when good stuff happens too, but beliefs and decisions made from good stuff are, obviously good for us. All these decisions and belief systems create our personalities.

I am about seven years old, and it is school report time – that dreaded time at the end of each term. What is it going to say this time? It doesn't matter because whatever it says, whatever grades I get, it will not be good enough.

One of my beliefs was I am not good enough; I am never good enough. This put a strain on me to keep trying hard because I needed the love and admiration that would result from being good enough, or this is what I told myself.

Deep down, I felt like a failure, but I didn't know this. I just kept failing, or did I? Or is this just the way I saw things from my "I'll never be good enough" position?

Whenever we have a belief system running, we filter out everything that doesn't support our beliefs. We can be the most successful person around and still believe we're not good enough.

How does this make us ill?

From the study of epigenetics (epi: above the gene), it is now known that genes are influenced by outside environmental signals. So, by changing the signal, it is possible to change the gene expression, and this, in turn, will change how your body functions.

Both Dr Bruce Lipton (*Biology of Belief*) and Dr Joe Dispenza (*Breaking the Habit of Being Yourself*) wrote about the effect of environmental factors on our bodies.

Our environment comprises our surroundings: the food we eat, the air we breathe—and our internal environment, which is constructed from the thoughts that arise from our belief systems. Change the way you think, and you change your internal environment—big time. Changing the way you think changes the way you feel.

"The concept that mind creates matter is not a metaphysical proposition. It's a biological one." – *Dawson Church,* Mind to Matter *2018*

Hay House, Inc., Carlsbad, CA

In a TED talk by Dr Alan Watkins, *"Being Brilliant Every Day,"* he explains how thoughts and feelings give rise to our performance. In a way, our disease is a performance—though you may not have thought of it that way. Your body is performing millions of processes all the time, and when you're ill, it produces horrid sensations.

So, if I can change the way I think, I can change my physiology. I can change the way I feel. I can change the way my body is performing.

I can do this in many ways, I can stop the stress responses by changing my beliefs, changing my breathing patterns, and using techniques like hypnosis or EFT. I can "see" my belief systems in a different way, I can "upgrade" my thinking. In a word, I can *change*.

Every time I integrated an unresolved issue, I changed. In the early days, I would get a lift followed by an upheaval, frequently referred to as a healing crisis. These were usually unpleasant but brief, and afterwards, I always felt better than I had before the integration.

As issues were resolved, other issues surfaced. At first, it felt like I was not improving and just getting other symptoms, but it was pointed out to me that the changes meant I was progressing, and that indeed proved to be the case.

I became more confident that I would heal through the process. Integration meant I was allowing my body to feel my emotions (e-motion=energy in motion), and as this processing continued, it freed up my energy. I was no longer using all of my energy to keep the traumas, the blocks in place. I had more and more energy for life. My emotions were moving through me, and therefore my energy was moving, so I could move.

One of the symptoms I experienced was a sort of heaviness of limb as if the air was thick or like moving through treacle. It was difficult to move, it took a lot of effort. My body was heavy, fatigued. I allowed myself to feel the emotion, and in this instance, it was despair—the despair of feeling trapped in an unsatisfying job. When I accepted this feeling, I gained a lot of energy.

In the end, I discovered that under it all, under all the negative and destructive feelings, were love, joy, and bliss.

May you be well

35

Resources

- Sedona Method: www.sedona.com
- The Journey: www.thejourneycom
- EFT/Tapping Technique: multiple sources online
- Havening Technique: Michele Paradise, Paul McKenna
- Meditation & Mindfulness Practices: See Chapter 14 on Meditation.
- Lifestyle Prescriptions: www.lifestyleprescriptions.org
- HeartMath: www.heartmath.org/heartmath.com
- The Chrysalis Effect: https://www.chrysaliseffecthealth.com/

Chapter 5: Spiritual or Energy Healing

I mentioned previously about the workshop on spiritual healing I had attended and that there had been two healers running it. I made an appointment to go and see one of them the following week. I chose the one who was also a qualified medical doctor, as his training in western medicine put me more at ease.

Unfortunately for me, he lived up two flights of stairs, so it took me a while to get to his office. I had to stop and rest several times on my way up.

Upon arriving and after a brief chat, I was asked to lie down on his treatment couch, and he moved his hands over me for about 20 to 30 minutes. I felt nothing.

After that, we chatted about my problems, my upbringing, and the idea of looking for answers within me. Although I had felt nothing, I arranged to go back the next week because, for the first time, I could talk about what was happening to me. He was someone who wanted to hear about my current problems and draw lines to how they were related to my past and my upbringing.

My childhood was not a happy one. My family was me, my parents, and an elder brother. I was born four years after the end of the Second World War, hence, finances were tight. My parents weren't happily married – a classic case of "marry in haste and repent at leisure." My father was an alcoholic and very irrational if he'd had too much to drink. I learned to be always on the alert for changes in his behaviour. I grew up never feeling safe, as there always seemed to be an underlying threat of violence— though this was usually verbal rather than physical.

Talking to this spiritual healer (I'll call him Michael) helped me understand how challenging this environment had been then and how it was affecting me now. Just being heard and accepted by Michael was a wonderful experience.

On the second visit, I was able to climb both flights of stairs in *one go*. What had happened?

To spiritual and energy healers, we are energy beings. Illness, symptoms, and pains are blocked energies or disharmonious energies left in place by unresolved trauma.

Energy healers and spiritual healers often see you as whole, well and recovered, and they use their abilities to move your energy and release the blockages to move you towards that wholeness.

Most would say they are the channel for the energy, that it is a natural phenomenon and that we all have the ability to release blockages. It has the essence of unconditional love. That love is a power, a force that can heal, and by using it, the body is helped to recognise its perfection. It helps us to get out of our own way.

38

The talking also helped as I was being heard. My negative beliefs in myself were being challenged. I was being given resources to move forward in my life.

I continued to see this healer for about six weeks, and at the last session, my hands and arms took on a life of their own. I was giving healing to him!

This experience was really curious. For a change, instead of lying down to receive, I was standing up, and as Michael moved his hands over me, suddenly I felt that I wanted to move. In fact, it was easier to let my arms move than hold them still, so I brought them up, and I could feel tingling in my hands as I held them towards Michael. I took this as a sign that I should train as a spiritual healer.

I went home and did some research on spiritual healing and found out about the Westcountry Natural Healing Fellowship. I contacted them and went on to training with them.

There was a wonderful woman who lived near my house. I used to go to her house with several other healers. Clients would come to her, and we would spend about 30 minutes with each person.

As we are channels for this healing energy, this unconditional love, we as healers get to benefit from it as well as it passes through us.

May you be free from pain

Resources

- Donna Eden – Energy Medicine:
  www.edenmethod.com
- Dr. Sue Morter: www.drsuemorter.com
- Dr. Eric Pearl: www.thereconnection.com
- Dr. Joe Dispenza: www.drjoedispenza.com
- Reiki: www.reiki.org

Chapter 6: Mind Works

One evening, I was fortunate enough to hear a talk by a hypnotherapist about her work in helping people heal themselves from numerous ailments. After the talk was over, I went up and asked if she could help me and made an appointment to go and see her.

But then, I became frightened of the idea of being hypnotised. When you have ME/CFS, you seem to be afraid of just about everything—I know I was.

I was on the verge of cancelling my appointment when I randomly heard a woman on the radio talking about her experience with hypnotherapy. She had been amazed by the results and had even used this approach to heal her piles!

Hearing this woman's account was a great comfort to me, and this sort of thing was becoming a regular occurrence in my life. I was receiving books to read and hear things that could be of help, and as I continued this healing path, these "signposts" became more obvious. If I heard, saw, or read something two to three times in quick succession, I took notice. It felt as if I was being guided.

I was reassured by this somewhat curious way of being spoken to by the universe and having my fears eased by this unknown person on the radio. It turned out that hypnotherapy was not only another major step in my recovery and discovering that my answers were within me, but over time, my therapist became a lifelong friend.

My therapist, I'll call her Wendy, took a detailed history and then explained exactly what would happen. It was easy, painless, and I didn't feel "out of it" at all. I was actually more aware and had easier access to memories.

During the history taking, I had described numerous symptoms, so she took one of those to work with during this session.

Wendy then hypnotised me by asking me to stare at a pointer which she held while she induced relaxation with guided imagery. Later, she gave me a recorded relaxation tape to use at home.

While deeply relaxed, she asked me when I had felt the sensations associated with the symptom previously in my life. In this relaxed state, I was easily able to recall a memory.

Although I can't remember now exactly what this memory was, it involved hiding behind a wall to protect myself. And I was still, in my unconscious mind, in hiding. While I was in this trance state, Wendy asked me whether I still needed this wall, was it still benefiting me or was there a drawback to its presence.

Wendy then asked me to suggest some resources that might be useful to me in this memory. Once I had named these resources and realised that I had them available to me, I understood that I didn't need the wall. But as the wall had been built when I was very young, Wendy advised me to just remove one course of bricks a day so that my emergence was gradual. I would gently adjust to the new state.

One reason memories remain a problem is that at the time of their formation, we were not resourceful, so we felt powerless and inadequate to deal with the situation. "Overwhelm" could be another way of describing the problem.

Because we couldn't deal with the event in a powerful way, we remain in that state and feel threatened, so we stay on high alert in case something similar happens. We become hypervigilant, unconsciously looking out for this to happen again. We feel the need to protect ourselves, and constantly being in this state is stressful and exhausting. Your adrenals are working overtime, secreting adrenaline and cortisol.

In a previous visit to a doctor, I discovered I was in this state during a knee-tap reflex test. The response was so strong that I nearly kicked him in the face. The doctor just laughed and didn't comment at all, but this really illustrated the high-stress state my body was in.

From about six sessions with Wendy, I developed my own system. I would push myself just a little bit, not too much, or I would be overwhelmed by illness and anxiety, but just enough so that I became aware of discomfort in my body. A balancing act, true, but with practice, I got good at it. I have learned to scan my body, to get "back into my body", to find what is trapped there, and to identify the trapped emotion(s). It's a skill well worth learning. With practice, I no longer needed to push myself past my comfort threshold.

As you can see, "my answers are within me." My body is speaking to me through my symptoms. I just need to stop, listen and learn. I still practice this as a form of meditation. I will explain this process in more detail in *Chapter 12: Learning to Body Scan*.

My life started to take on new meaning, as I was no longer bothered about recovery. I was exploring life, how it works, my past, who I was and who or what I am now—and recovery was simply *happening*. No longer was I being driven by fear, but instead, led by curiosity. What joy!

I have also trained as a "Journey Therapist" with Brandon Bays—though I don't practice now. A "*Journey*" process is an amazing tool for uncovering past trauma and healing the body.

That all came about because I was given the book *The Journey* before it had been released into bookshops—another significant signpost. It's worth pointing out that I don't follow up on everything that happens in this way. Discernment is required! Usually, though, it's sound guidance.

During my training, I decided to do a session on the memory for my ME/CFS and where it was stored in my body. The process started with a brief guided meditation, and my internal guidance took me to my hypothalamus. Now, this was fascinating to me as the hypothalamus is involved with regulating the homeostatic systems in the body, keeping the various systems in balance.

I will unpack this!

Homeostasis is the body's ability to self-regulate through various feedback pathways. It is how the body keeps itself comfortable and in balance, and one of the experiences of ME/CFS is that our bodies do not feel comfortable. Homeostasis means '*same state.*'

The hypothalamus is responsible for, among other things: body temperature, hunger, fatigue and sleep. It also controls parts of the pituitary gland, so it has a major role in the endocrine system as well.

The memory that arose was when a practical joke by a few school friends went seriously wrong. I, along with my other co-victims, thought we were going to be killed, and I believed we had to fight for our lives.

It is our last year of school, and six of us, three girls and three boys, decide to rent a cottage on Exmoor, a national park in Devon, England. It's very remote, in a forest, with no electricity.

On the third night, some of the other students from school decide to come out and visit us. During the evening, someone suggests holding a séance—they were all the rage back then! I absolutely don't want to do this, but as I am in the minority, the ritual rolls ahead.

Using an upside-down glass and a board with letters on it, questions are asked. Who knows who or what was moving it, but the glass moves as if inhabited by a spirit. And what "it," says isn't friendly.

After this, our visitors leave. Five of us walk them back to their cars, and one boy stays behind. We get a bit lost in the dark and end up walking across a marshy area where the ground is very soggy and soft. For some reason, our flashlights stop working, all of them. So, with the other students going, there are five of us in complete darkness, needing to find our way back. The tension is high and rising.

We set off down the farm track leading to our cottage, and then...something starts following us. We can't see clearly in the dark, but it appears to be an amorphous shape with red glowing "eyes." I want to go and investigate, but the boys aren't up for that.

It keeps following us, we can hear it, and then two of us get separated from the other three. We hear a girl scream.

By now, the two of us had got back to the cottage, and I tried the door, but it was locked. This thing keeps coming. I hear it tramping over the ground towards us. I am terrified, and my friend is cowering behind me. I am trapped between the cottage and this thing—there is no escape, I have to confront it. Holding the torch as a weapon, I say, "If you come any closer, I'll kill you."

It stops and morphs into the boy that had stayed behind. Apparently, I had called his name (I don't remember doing so) because he replies, "Oh, you knew who it was all the time."

No, *I think* I hadn't known. *If I had, I wouldn't have been terrified.*

For some reason, they had wanted to frighten me, and they were very successful. What have I done to merit this? I am angry, then deeply hurt.

After, none of us girls can sleep. We need to keep the light on. As the "jokers" are our friends, very little is said, either at the time or afterwards.

It wasn't so long after this that I started with irregular heartbeats but never made the connection. At the time, I didn't know there might be one.

May you be free from fear

Resources

There are many tools and techniques available to help in rewriting our personal history, discover our own answers, and change our experience of life. Here are some of the ones I used.

- The Journey with Brandon Bays: www.thejourney.com
- The Work (app) - Byron Katie: https://thework.com
- Hypnotherapy
- Counseling
- Meditation
- Meta-Health: metahealthacademy.com
- Meta-Kinetics
- Lifestyle Prescriptions: lifestyleprescriptions.org
- The Chrysalis Effect: https://www.chrysaliseffecthealth.com/
- As our programming is also stored in the body I include:
- Massage especially Myofascial Release (MFR)
- Yoga
- Tai Chi
- Acupuncture
- Alexander Technique
- Sound therapy

- Bio-energetics: Dr. Sue Morter

Books

- *The Journey* by Brandon Bays
- *The Untrue Story of You* by Bryan Hubbard
- *The Healing Power of Illness: Understanding What Your Symptoms Are Telling You* by Thorwald Dethlefsen and Rüdiger Dalhke
- *Molecules of Emotion* by Candace Pert
- *The Biology of Belief* by Dr. Bruce Lipton
- *The Body Keeps the Score* by Bessel van der Kolk
- *Loving What Is* by Byron Katie
- *Waking the Tiger* by Peter Levine
- *In an Unspoken Voice* by Peter Levine
- *Trauma Through a Child's Eyes* by Peter Levine
- *Mind to Matter* by Dawson Church
- *Cured* by Dr. Jeff Rediger

Why do these therapies work?

These therapies help you to become resourceful in situations where you weren't, so the body relaxes. It, you, cease to need to be hypervigilant. You are no longer being confronted and threatened by past traumas and inner demons.

Chapter 7: The Effects of Negative Childhood Experiences

I recently listened to a talk by a paediatrician where I learned about the research into "Adverse Childhood Experiences" (A.C.E.s) and the effects they have on our adult behaviour. I learned that children with traumatic childhoods are far more likely to develop heart disease, cancer, etc., and die at a younger age. Our adulthood can be a persistent state of PTSD as we try to recover from and make sense of our initial experiences!

The paediatrician reported that to a child, the absence of a caring person is highly damaging. This is especially the case for a child living with an adult that has, for example, substance abuse, anger issues, or is neglectful. Why is something that happened so long ago still affecting us? Why do childhood issues make us ill?

Fortunately, there is now a lot of research into the phenomenon of previous trauma causing present-day problems. It's obvious that trauma causes mental and emotional issues—sadly, we see that with many of our soldiers, hospital workers, police, etc. They are diagnosed with PTSD, which is deemed to be a mental and emotional problem. But what if physical diseases are also a form of PTSD?

All the feelings that you are experiencing are felt in your body. Your mind is causing your body to produce various chemical and electrical signals which are produced in the body, by the body, and which affect the body.

See something scary, and your body goes into flight or fight mode? If you get habituated to being in this state because of work pressure or because of your own thoughts, you get stuck in fight, flight, or freeze.

Our sympathetic nervous system is set up to ensure that we survive. That is its purpose, and it takes priority over everything else. We move away from pain far faster than we move toward pleasure. We are hard-wired to do so. I remember hearing that this response is ten times stronger, so we're truly up against it.

It's vital that it's set up this way, it does save our lives. However, if we suffer persistent attacks on our physical, mental or emotional well-being as children, we will be on the lookout (unconsciously) for it as adults. We can interpret the slightest negative comment or situation as extremely threatening to our well-being. And so, we remain in a constant state of stress, secreting adrenaline and cortisol because we are trying to escape or preparing to fight. Or we simply freeze and "play dead."

But as children in persisting adverse situations, there was no escape. There was nowhere to go. Our caregivers were maybe even the ones threatening us, so we were in a bind. We were completely dependent on the one attacking us. This gave us mixed messages.

As I said before, my father was a class act at giving mixed messages. Apart from not knowing how he was going to react, he was also always threatening to abandon us. And the mixed message I was giving myself was that I still loved him despite all of this.

This constant hypervigilance for signs of rejection, criticism, or shame is stressful and exhausting, and because it is happening all day, every day, it becomes normalised. No wonder I felt so free when I went off to Girl Guide camp.

Living in this state will also lead to adrenal exhaustion. Our adrenals are supposed to be on standby for emergency use, not on constant duty.

We, as children, felt that something was seriously wrong, but we didn't have the resources to understand *what*. If we couldn't run away, we were likely to go into the third response of the autonomic (automatic) nervous system (ANS), and that is to shut down or freeze.

If I were to liken my experience to a computer program, I would say I was running malware. My software (my beliefs) was not functioning for my benefit and health, and contradictory programs were causing all sorts of malfunctions (diseases). And so, I discovered I needed to upgrade my programming.

It has been said that it's never too late to have a happy childhood. Of course, you can't change your childhood experiences, but you can release yourself from their legacy. As my cousin, an inspirational teacher, was to say, "Don't let your past destroy your future." In that way, whatever our childhood was like (and some are a lot grimmer than mine), we can free ourselves to be happy and healthy. If we don't do the work, not only do we stay trapped in the past for fear of repeating these experiences, but we continually relive them in the present through conditioning.

I remember performing an exercise on a retreat that involved having an imaginary sack into which we put our traumas, issues, and problems as we walked around. After just a few minutes, I couldn't move and just sat down by a chair on the floor, feeling exhausted. I didn't even sit on the chair, just made myself as small and as hidden as possible.

I was weighed down by the unresolved issues that I was carrying. Does that feel like something you might have experienced?

Another therapy I learned at this retreat was Family Constellations. This is an amazing process for healing our past and is done in groups.

The person whose issue is being addressed picks group members to represent the people relevant to the issue and places them in the room. It seems unnecessary for much guidance to be given to the "actors" for this process to work. Then the person whose issue is being addressed sits down to watch what happens. And something does; somehow, the actors know what to do, say, and where to move.

It's astonishing being both an actor and an observer because everyone seems to gain benefit.

It is my turn, and I pick just one other person. He is just standing where I placed him, and I am feeling threatened, and I am cowering away, shouting "No, no, no," over and over again. I back away, still repeating no. Suddenly, there is a shift in my body, and I start to feel strong and powerful. I straighten and stand up. I walk slowly and steadily, holding and owning my power. I look at this person, and I stare them down, and they crumble.

I didn't know who the person was. All I needed to know was I had access to this power. I did not need to hold on to smallness and powerlessness.

Not all negative incidents will result in illness. There are many examples of people having the most horrendous experiences without lasting problems. They seem to have an innate resilience, or is it a learned response? Maybe both. But it is certainly possible to learn resilience.

Meta-Health and Lifestyle Prescriptions are approaches that focus on body/mind/social health with an understanding that certain emotions and adverse events are organ-specific. For example, if you have an abandonment trauma, the epidermis of the skin is the affected organ. According to the Meta-Health and Lifestyle Prescriptions paradigm, there do seem to be certain characteristics of types of trauma that make it more likely to be damaging.

· It is unexpected

· It is dramatic

· It is isolating

· It is frequently contrary to our belief system

I am nine years old. I believe I am helping a friend out, but our actions are disapproved of by a teacher who tells us to go and stand away from our friends and in front of the rest of the girls in the dining hall (about 80 pupils). This teacher had always treated me as a bit of a favourite as her brother was my father's boss.

She shouts at us from the other side of the hall, telling us we are sly and deceitful.

This episode fulfils all the above criteria:

- I am experiencing fear and shame and would like to disappear.

- It felt overwhelming.

- I am separated from my peers.

- It was completely unexpected and contrary to my belief that, because she had treated me well in the past, she would treat me that way this time.

Much later, when I got around to releasing this episode, I discovered I was experiencing a whole lot more.

- An ache in the left arm
- Tension
- Fear of speaking up
- Fear of confrontation
- Contempt for teachers/authority figures
- Fear of betrayal
- Avoiding any situation that had even the slightest potential to be similar
- Rage
- Injustice
- Resentment
- Shame

I wasn't aware that I was in this state at all, but it was taking a toll on my physical body. I was secreting cortisol and adrenaline.

I believe that when I originally became ill, I had run out of psychic energy, which I was using to suppress all these very unpleasant sensations. All my negative experiences, with all their accompanying feelings and emotions, could no longer be repressed, and they all burst out at once and became my illness—which was an overwhelming experience in itself.

I discovered that I had a lot of repressed anger, though because it was repressed, I was unaware that it was anger. I was experiencing it as fear instead. There is a lot of energy in anger, and it takes an equal amount to repress it. The energy I needed for simply living wasn't available to me.

According to American physician and psychiatrist Alexander Lowen, we can hold these feelings in by something called muscular armouring. We tense our muscles in order not to feel, and this muscular holding is very tiring. Whether we are moving our muscles or holding them, we are using energy.

When I didn't know what my father was going to do or what I should do, my body would go into freeze mode. I was too small to fight (I would certainly lose), and I had nowhere safe to run to. Freezing was the best and most logical way my unconscious survival mechanism found to cope—if I didn't do anything, nothing bad could happen.

And I would like to shout this out loud: IT IS NOT MY/YOUR FAULT THAT YOU/I ARE ILL! We/you are not deliberately creating our illness. I/you just didn't have the help, the resources to handle our experiences. But I took responsibility, and when I did that, I started to find ways to recover.

When memories get stored, they store everything, all the things you are aware of and all the things you are not aware of:

- The clothes – people, including you, are wearing.
- The sounds – what was said, what was heard (such as cars braking, people shouting).
- Where did it happen?
- What were you feeling?
- The decisions you made at the time: *I'm powerless, I'm not safe, and I'm shameful.* Smells and tastes.
- Where it happened
- What you were feeling

Because so much of this is not in our conscious awareness, if we meet any one of these factors in the present time, we can be triggered. As we are unaware of the connection, our bodily reactions can be bizarre and therefore frightening, adding more stress and anxiety. Making the connection and remembering (remember: to join up again, to make the connection) can be healing in itself.

Before I got ill, I was a reasonably relaxed flyer, not that I did much. Afterwards, I became almost phobic. I could fly, but I was tense, wanted to cry, my teeth would chatter, and I always felt that I might die.

When I was about seven years old, I had my tonsils removed in hospital which was quite a bad experience for me.

The connection that my unconscious mind had made was the long narrow shape of the aircraft with the long, narrow shape of the ward where frightening things happened. And even though I came out of the hospital, my fear and anxiety remained buried within me.

As an adult and knowing this, I can separate then from now. I have released the trigger.

And so, I discovered that my symptoms were mainly unresolved childhood incidents.

Frequently, just knowing the traumas of one's childhood and seeing them from an adult's perspective can be healing. You, as an adult, know what you needed at the time. As my first healer said, "All your answers are within you."

But sometimes, this is not enough.

May you be well

Resources: See Chapter 6

Chapter 8: Discovery: The Power of Forgiveness to Heal

Why should I forgive them? They shouldn't have done this to me. They're to blame; it's not my fault.

Forgiveness sets *us* free. It releases us from the past. It opens us up to the present, to be here *now*. If we live in the now, then our past traumas cannot affect us. We are free— free of past conditioning, of being triggered, and free to live joyously and spontaneously.

The "perpetrator" probably doesn't give a damn. They may not even have thought they had "wronged" you or given it a second thought since it happened

It happened; wishing it hadn't is natural, but it did. If it hasn't been forgiven and released for you, it is still happening, right here, right now. By holding onto the grievance and the resentment, you keep yourself locked in the past. And in this case, the painful past.

Just look at the word "re-sent-ment." Who is resending this to you time and time again? Who is re-feeling this? You are, I was. I honestly thought I was punishing the perpetrators for the pain they caused me, and it was a *big* wake-up call to find that I was punishing myself.

Feelings of anger and resentment poison our bodies: these angry and resentful thoughts cause us stress, so we secrete cortisol and adrenaline. Excess cortisol secretion can lead to high blood pressure, tension, bad digestion, etc. These feelings may cause us to lose sleep and have bad dreams. It's now well-known that stress is a major contributor to ill health, so why add to it by holding onto anger and resentment?

Holding on keeps us in the flight, fight or freeze mode because, as far as we're concerned, it's still happening. Another good reason to forgive and let go.

Forgiveness is not always easy to find, especially if you tell yourself it "shouldn't have happened." Maybe it shouldn't, but it has, and "getting over it" is not always possible without help.

There are times when I have been seriously unkind and said things I later regretted. But why? Because that moment, I was in pain, so I can assume that the people who hurt me are/were also in pain. The more I let go of my wounds, the more my heart opens to all, and the more that I can accept all. The more I cannot be hurt or shamed, the more resilient to stress I become. I lose my knee-jerk reactions to potentially stressful situations.

I haven't worked out if these situations don't arise anymore or if I simply don't notice them. I do notice that people get upset over inconsequential things, and I'm curious. Did I use to be reactive like that?

Forgiveness: to give up and to allow.

Just think of someone you haven't forgiven; how do you feel in your body? Do you feel tight, hard, or resistant? Where in your body do you feel it? Does your body feel comfortable?

Now think of someone you love or a pet you would always forgive. See how you feel now. Now think: how forgiving of yourself are you? Do you feel love and kindness toward yourself?

True forgiveness is a felt sense, a visceral and somatic experience. It does not occur only in the mind.

What if you absolutely can't forgive?

We have all had experiences that we would probably prefer not to have had, including some seriously bad experiences. But it's probably true to say that what doesn't kill you can make you stronger. If you can transcend and integrate the experience, you grow. Your heart will be a little bit more open.

People who are hurt and wounded hurt other people, and so the pain carries on. Maybe now is the time to stop this destructive pattern in our own lives, our families, our towns and villages, and even our countries.

As I have said, my father was an alcoholic, which caused him to be erratic and unpredictable. And I hated that. Of course, as a child, I couldn't understand, but as an adult, taking a step back, I know that it wasn't a lifestyle choice. It was his way of dealing with his pain. We all adopt habits and addictions to comfort ourselves, so am I going to condemn someone, withhold forgiveness from someone, or myself, because of the pain they and I are feeling?

"Judge softly," Mary T. Lathrapp

"Walk a mile in their moccasins," American Indian proverb.

The Journey with Brandon Bays is an awesome forgiveness process. So is *Loving What Is*, by Byron Katy. *The Journey* is the author's guide to how she healed herself through forgiveness and *Loving What Is* is a way of challenging our beliefs and getting past our resistance to what happened, allowing us to let go and move on. I found these amazing tools for getting over the stories I was telling myself about what I had experienced.

Try forgiving a little and see how good it feels. Maybe increase that amount. If you can't forgive, seek help. Just saying, "I forgive" is not sufficient (though it's a very good start), as it's a felt thing, and simply giving lip service doesn't set us free.

Try writing a letter to them—you won't send it, so it doesn't matter what you write. And do it on paper as you are going to burn it afterwards.

Keep forgiving. Maybe try saying something like, "it is love that forgives through me."

Try Ho'ponopono (Hawaiian Forgiveness Mantra: I love you, I'm sorry, forgive me). This is a good practice if you find it difficult to forgive—somehow, it just works.

I have found that events can have many aspects, and they all need my forgiveness.

Forgiving someone does not mean condoning the action. It may remain appalling and even unforgivable (now there's a paradox) but the damaged, hurt human perpetrator is forgivable, and that includes you. You, too, need your own love and forgiveness.

Work through your "list" of people and events that need your forgiveness. This may take some time! You will know whether it is complete by how you feel in your body. Be gentle with yourself. Some things do seem impossible to allow and accept—get help if you need it.

The more I forgave, the more I released, the freer I became, the more I recovered, the more accepting I became, the less I judged good and bad, and the more my heart opened. It's still a work in progress. It probably always will be.

Seeing someone's behaviour from a more open and loving heart may help you more easily forgive what happened in the past. Understanding that they were doing the best they could at the time (even if that wasn't good at all) has also helped me to let go.

Forgiving the past also brings you into the present, where true change and freedom can occur.

I may always judge other people's actions and behaviours, but I don't need to hang onto them. As I notice them arise—from someone cutting me up in traffic, someone letting a door go in my face, even me being a bit short with my husband—I work through why I am feeling the way I am and then forgive; myself, them, and anyone else.

And a paradox occurs when, ultimately, one finds that there is nothing to forgive. When you can forgive, deeply and totally, everyone who has ever hurt you or wronged you, including yourself, you are free to see them as they are, hurt and maybe damaged human beings, just like you, doing the best that they can at the time. Am I really going to judge anyone like this?

And now, I need to discover the questions to know what is within me.

May you be happy

Resources

The Journey by Brandon Bays

The Sedona Method

Institute of HeartMath practices

Ho'ponopono (Hawaiian Forgiveness Mantra: I love you, I'm sorry, forgive me)

Loving What Is by Byron Katy

EFT

Chapter 9: The Power of Self-Inquiry

As I have said, the first healer I had repeatedly told me that "all my answers are within me," from which I inferred that I needed to ask myself relevant questions. But what is a "relevant question?" And what is the benefit of finding your own answers?

Some people are more resourceful and resilient than others, but you can learn to be more resourceful and resilient (see HeartMath). You can raise your threshold from someone who reacts badly to everything to someone who takes most of life in stride. Believe me, I've done both. Life is much more comfortable that way and infinitely more enjoyable.

It's no one's fault. You are simply being triggered into feelings and behaviours that originated when you were very small and didn't have access to the tools and resources you can now access.

If you raise your tolerance level for difficulties, you will not notice them. I haven't decided whether the trauma I have integrated doesn't happen anymore or if I don't notice when it does.

I know when something is completely integrated because all emotional charge has gone. It's almost as if it didn't happen or it happened to someone else—which is true. I was someone else then.

These days I frequently have an inner dialogue. As soon as I notice a somatic reaction, I investigate. Something has triggered this response, and if it's a negative response that increases my stress reaction, I don't want it. I want to resolve it as soon as possible so that I may return to a state of well-being and peacefulness.

How do I know to do/feel this sensation?

If I'm doing something, whatever it is, whether I'm being afraid, jealous, angry, feeling a knot in my stomach, the tension in my jaw or shoulders, pain in my back or anywhere, I know how to do it—not *why* I am doing it. But asking myself why I am doing something opens me up to telling myself a story, and that's not necessarily a particularly constructive approach.

How do I know to be angry? Somewhere, at some time, I felt deprived and hurt. Is that my experience now? Yes, it is because I'm feeling that, but is it true in the current circumstances—and even if it is, can I let it go? Does this feeling serve me? What would I prefer to experience?

What stops the love from flowing, that feeling of deep peace and well-being?

It is my responsibility; I can change my feeling and experience even if the initial "knee jerk" reaction is anger or fear. Noticing and becoming aware of the response means I now have a choice. Stuff happens and will always happen; how I respond is my choice.

Freedom does not prevent feeling triggered or even prevent being afraid of being triggered but accepts all that is arising.

I found I had to get real. I was seriously angry but expressing anger as a child was, to put it bluntly, dangerous. So, what did I do with it? I suppressed it, numbed out and developed all sorts of muscular armouring not to feel it. My body was much stiffer than it is today because I've released a lot of it. I can't say all of it because how do I know?

When I first came across my anger, it frightened me.

I am walking my dog on nearby common land, and suddenly I feel overwhelmed by rage. It's so strong I think I'm going to die. There is this inner demon, a witch-like female, and I feel that if I'm going to survive, I need to put her in a cage. By doing this, the anger eases. I have regained control and some equanimity.

I have no idea what triggered this. Maybe it was simply time for me to deal with some of my anger.

All that energy was tied up inside me. Bit by bit, using whatever technique helped at the moment allowed me to integrate it. But it happened over time and not all at once.

I used EFT, mindfulness, and body scanning—and sometimes, I would have to deal with it later when I had a quiet moment. This would happen when I would participate in boxing. The first time I sparred with anyone, I was amazed at the peace I felt after boxing for less than five minutes. A deep letting go, a deep tranquillity, a deep sense of freedom.

What's the story I'm telling myself about this situation?

If I'm suffering, I resist what is happening, probably saying something like, "it shouldn't have happened." "Well, it did, get over it," is far too crude and unhelpful—we would have got over it if we could. But just looking at the very idea that I'm telling myself a story helps to distance myself from it and bring in more perspectives. Stuff happens, and we don't like a lot of it, but bad stuff can help us grow.

What's the benefit of being ill?

This is a challenging question, but it's well worth asking. A secondary gain of being ill was that I didn't have to go to work at a job that I found completely unfulfilling. This led me to accept that I was in the wrong job.

My mother had always pressured me into finding a career in case my future marriage didn't work out. She was influenced by her experience of being stuck in an unsatisfactory relationship. So, I had opted for physiotherapy, and once in it, it felt wrong, but with a mortgage and other financial commitments, I felt trapped. I needed the money, so I kept doing it.

There will be reasons, valid reasons for you to unearth. It takes total honesty with yourself (no one else needs to know). It also takes understanding and compassion. And it may be easier to start with, to look at any resistance to recovering. I found quite a bit of resistance in the beginning. I was afraid my increased energy would be consumed by mundane tasks such as housework and other duties and chores. Who would want to get better just to do the ironing?

Once you know what you *don't* want, you can move towards finding something that gives meaning and purpose to your life, that lights you up, and brings pleasure and satisfaction.

Another benefit was using my illness to avoid situations that made me feel uncomfortable or that I didn't want to do. I was able to control not only myself but other people as well. I realised I hadn't the courage to say no, so I felt (more) ill instead. Remember that this is totally out of one's conscious awareness until you make it conscious. No blame, no judgment, no self-condemnation, simply self-acceptance of the only tool I had to control the overwhelm I was experiencing.

My life as a child had been chaotic and challenging, and my life at the time of the onset was full of issues—I was using this illness to avoid both. In the end, I have chosen to face my demons so that I no longer live a half-life.

71

Other questions often asked.

"Who/what/where am I?"

This can be done as an exercise with someone else. If you choose to do it with a partner, get them to ask you the question "who are you?" and when you reply, they then say thank you and repeat the question, "who are you?" and continue for as long as you like or until you can't come up with an answer. Or simply ask yourself that same question. Here is an example:

Who am I? – Jill – thank you

Who am I?- I'm a woman – thank you

Who am I?- I'm a physio – thank you

Who am I? – I don't know – thank you

Who am I? – somebody (some body) – thank you

Who am I? – nobody (no body) – thank you

Who am I – peacefulness – thank you

Who am I? – pure potentiality – thank you

You can continue to question for a set time limit or until there is silence.

What's the worst thing that can happen? And if that happens, what is the worst thing that can happen? And if that.....?

Is it true?

What am I feeling?

Where in my body am I feeling it?

When have I felt like this before? And before that? And before that? If there is a root cause, what is it? If there is a core event...?

Is this "old stuff" coming up?

What is stopping my love from flowing?

May you be at peace

Resources

HeartMath:

www.heartmath.org or www.heartmath.com

Loving What Is and *The Work* - Byron Katy www.thework.com

The Journey – www.thejourney.com

Neuro-linguistic Programming (NLP) – many online resources

EFT www.dawsonchurch.com tapping technique, etc

Bio-Energetics - Dr Sue Morter

Sedona Method – www.sedonamethod.com

Mindfulness – mindful.org and many other online sources

Chapter 10: The Power of Correct Breathing

So far, I have concentrated on the mind so let's move on to the body. Our feelings, aches and pains are stored and felt here, and just as it's "never too late to have a happy childhood," it's also not too late to have a comfortable body. The more you release, the more delicious to be in your body becomes.

I was recently sitting in a concert, and I noticed that the three people in front of me raised their shoulders every time they breathed in. I started to look around and was amazed at how many people were doing this.

It's so important to breathe *properly*—is it really that complicated? It shouldn't be. It's the first obvious thing we do at birth and the last thing we do as we die, yet most of us don't appear to do it very well. Even if you can't do much because of ME/CFS, you can at least breathe well!

One of the first things you can do to start is breathing through your nose. Simply doing this creates huge benefits—I encourage you to read *Breath* by James Nestor to learn more.

Secondly, learn to breathe deep in your chest. As a physiotherapist, part of my job was to check patients' chests and breathing pre-and post-op and to make sure they could and would cough to prevent post-operative chest infections. I often found many patients were not breathing well and deeply—they were not using their diaphragms much, if at all. It's a natural process over which we have a little control—we can hold our breath, breathe into different parts of our chest, and change the rhythm and frequency. So why are so many of us not breathing properly?

The fact that healthy babies do breathe well offers a clue. One of the reasons we don't breathe properly as adults is because of stored trauma in the body, causing us stress.

When something bad is happening, we will go into flight or fight mode and start to breathe more quickly so that we can flee or fight. We are now cortisol- and adrenaline-dominant and stressed. If the issue is not resolved and integrated or accepted, we remain stressed. This may become such a normal feeling that we cease to be aware of when it is happening. Then it becomes a problem.

One of the many diagnoses I received initially was hyperventilation syndrome. In other words, I was breathing far too quickly at rest, so it was probably not surprising that I was having attacks of dizziness, tachycardia (rapid heart rate) and panic. This was evidence that I was stressed, but to be honest, before I became ill, if someone had asked me, I would have said I was OK! I thought I was coping. I had no idea I was being affected by my past.

We might breathe too quickly, but when in pain, physical or mental, we tend to hold our breath.

Changing the way that we breathe and where in our chests, we can have profound and lasting effects on our health and well-being. We can change how we feel by changing the way that we breathe. We can also breathe to alleviate both physical and emotional or mental pain.

The breath cycle (an in-breath and an out-breath is one cycle) affects our autonomic nervous system (ANS). I often hear people tell someone feeling anxious or nervous to take a deep breath, but that may actually be counterproductive. Taking a deep breath usually means that people inflate the upper part of their chest, thereby stimulating the sympathetic (flight, fight, freeze) branch of the ANS, leading to more tension and anxiety rather than less.

In order to calm down, the practice of breathing in and out has to be equal in length. Balancing the two branches of the autonomic nervous system or the out-breath can be slightly longer. For example, breathe in and out and count to five or in for five and out for seven or eight. Your breathing should never feel strained or cause breathlessness when you want to feel relaxed, so adjust my suggestions to suit you.

As we breathe in, the sympathetic branch is excited, and as we breathe out, the parasympathetic (rest, digest, and heal) branch is affected. So, if we want to relax, we need to become parasympathetic dominant—making the out-breath slightly longer.

Breathwork is also a major part of some meditation practices, but you do not need to sit in meditation to work on your breathing. It does take practice to change your breathing habits and carry them over into everyday life. In the beginning, I would practice several times a day. As I recovered, I would notice my breath patterns when stopped at traffic lights, in a supermarket queue, anywhere—until my default breathing pattern was parasympathetic-dominant.

HeartMath, an American research institute with branches in the UK, South Africa, and Australia, has been studying the effects of different breathing patterns in humans for years. They have written many peer-reviewed papers on breathing, and something referred to as heart rate variability (HRV) and have used this data to develop an app. There are also other apps you can use to monitor your breath.

Having what is known as a coherent HRV is very good for your health. HRV is the naturally occurring beat-to-beat changes in heart rate and a coherent HRV, in lay terms, means your body is functioning optimally.

An optimal level of HRV within an organism reflects healthy function and an inherent self-regulatory capacity, adaptability and resilience.

From the HeartMath Institute

If you can establish a coherent HRV, then your body starts to secrete a hormone called dehydroepiandrosterone (DHEA). This is a hormone of healing. It also has other beneficial effects, such as slowing the signs of ageing! It is also the opposite of the stress hormone cortisol, so the more DHEA you are secreting, the less cortisol you will have and the more you are in the parasympathetic (rest, digest, and heal) mode.

The correct way of breathing, accompanied by a positive emotion such as appreciation, results in a whole cocktail of feel-good hormones being secreted. Feel-good hormones do what they say—they make us feel good.

You can see whether you're breathing deep in your chest or shallowly by placing your hand on your upper chest and the other below your ribs on your abdomen. Your lower hand should rise and fall as your abdomen expands, and your upper hand should stay still. If this isn't happening, put some time into learning the proper technique.

Sometimes it is very difficult for people to get the right pattern. Try breathing out and pulling in your tummy first and then relax and let in the air. If that doesn't work, try pushing down a bit on the seat of your chair. And see if that helps.

Always breathe through the nose unless your nose is bunged up. Breathing through the nose reduces the chance of hyperventilation (over-breathing) which can induce panic attacks. I have also found that it has virtually eliminated the odd irregular heartbeat I used to have.

What exactly does breathing do for us? It gets rid of carbon dioxide. It supplies oxygen to the body. It's a valuable tool for centring. Correctly done, it can change our state. It can bring emotional balance. It can be a focus for meditation.

Yogis and other cultures have developed different breathing exercises for different purposes (pranayama). We now have the science to observe and measure what these various types of practices can do for us.

When in physical or emotional pain, balanced breathing will help to alleviate the issue. It will help to dispel negative and blocked emotions stored in the body. By breathing as if through the blockage, the pain, the sensations, and energy can then begin to move, relax and dissipate.

This has been mostly about balancing the autonomic nervous system to calm us, but there are many other breathing techniques to try. Some of these can help to bring buried emotions to the surface: holotropic breathing (developed by Stan Grof), cyclic breathing, rebirthing, etc. These practices are extremely powerful and need to be done under expert guidance.

Holotropic breathing is a method where you breathe rapidly and without pausing between the in-breath and the out-breath. It can induce an altered state to access past trauma—and a deeper understanding of oneself.

I did a holotropic breath session while on retreat. After about 20 or more minutes of nothing much happening, a voice in my head declared, "you're a sham." I just started laughing, and laughing, and laughing, and…fortunately, I was already lying down because I rolled around the floor completely and totally lost in this laughter which went on and on for over an hour.

What a release—and what a happy way of doing it! Everything was funny for the next 24 to 36 hours, and I felt glorious. I started to come down after that, which was just as well as I had to drive home.

This reaction would not necessarily happen if I did another holotropic breathwork session (and as I haven't found anywhere close to me, I haven't repeated it), but it was wonderful at the time. It was also a sign that I was recovering, as my sense of humour returned.

May you be well.

Resources

Institute of HeartMath – www.heartmath.org

Central Channel Breathing - Dr Sue Morter, the Morter Institute

Transformational Breath transformationalbreath.com Alternate Nostril Breathing - see yoga practices.

Breath by James Nestor

Holotropic Breathing – www.holotropic.com

Omnibreath – www.omnibreath.com

Apps

Inner Balance

HeartBreath

Breath Pacer

Chapter 11: Getting Physical – Learning to Feel

The title of this chapter may seem a bit odd. We're feeling all the time and usually, like sh…

As I've already mentioned, I view chronic fatigue as what takes over when we tire of maintaining our great resistance to feeling emotions. For most of us ME/CFS feels like running a marathon with flu—a pretty accurate description.

Learning to feel can be very scary. After all, we numbed out for a reason—a type of avoidance. Confronting what we trained ourselves to avoid and re-establishing connection with past trauma needs to be done carefully and perhaps with expert help.

As I have said, I used alcohol and cigarettes to numb out, and both of those crutches were taken away from me. I distinctly remember the last time I smoked. I was leaving Dartmouth, Devon, on our boat and had lit a cigarette. I took one puff, felt even worse than usual, flicked the rest of the cigarette over the side and never smoked again. The pain outweighed the pleasure. And by this time, even half a glass of wine made my heart race until the alcohol was out of my system. Without my crutches, I was left to feel everything—and in this state, the feelings were intense.

When I was ill, it was as if my body had a mind of its own. If I pushed it too far (no matter what I did), it reacted, and I didn't seem able to stop it because I didn't understand what was happening. This was terrifying. Walking too quickly or climbing stairs a bit quickly would trigger tachycardia that might go on for hours.

I was doing well in my recovery from ME/CFS by using my mind, but somehow my body was lagging. So what did I want from physical approaches? I wanted to get the tension out of my body, I wanted to "get into my body", and I wanted to continue to release the trauma stored in my body. I wanted to learn to feel.

I did loads of different things to see what worked best for me, using myself as a research tool.

Observing your breath, feeling the air pass through your nose, its quality (moist or dry), how your chest moves and so on is a simple and effective way of gaining body awareness and learning to feel. It's such an integral part of the process that I've given it its own chapter (Twelve: Learning to Body Scan) but read on here for some other ways to learn how to feel.

There are therapies like a massage that are done to us rather than us doing them ourselves. They also help to get our energy moving.

<u>Massage</u>

If you like being touched, then massage is for you. Being touched on the outside helps to reawaken us to our bodies' presence and reduce the numbing. Many of us, as little children, didn't have that comforting touch that we needed to feel safe, nurtured and loved.

Find a therapist that will massage you in the way that you like. This is very important, as some of us like a soft touch and others a firmer touch. Either way, you'll need to find someone who is decisive and confident with their touch, as tentativeness and diffidence will only make you tenser. We need to feel held, safe and protected.

There are so many different types of massage, so it's also crucial to figure out what type will help you best. When I learned how to be a physiotherapist, we worked in Swedish massage. This method involves long, sweeping strokes over the body. Incorporating essential oils turns it into aromatherapy, with some scents used for relaxation and others being more stimulating.

There is also Thai massage, Indian head massage, Lomi Lomi massage, Myofascial Release, Rolfing, etc. The beneficial effects are legion—if you like being touched, that is. Deepak Chopra has been known to say that if we could bottle the beneficial effects of massage and then *not* give it to our patients, we would be guilty of malpractice.

If you don't like being touched because of trauma or any other reason, you can massage yourself with oils or creams or try Havening. I love Havening, especially when an issue arises, as it immediately calms me. It involves stroking the upper arms as if hugging yourself, changing your brainwaves from high beta (stressed) to a more relaxed delta frequency. Havening can be used for releasing trauma both in the present and the past.

Massage or any therapy involving appropriate touch helps put you back in contact with your body. The outside stimulus helps you feel your body in a comforting and enjoyable way.

Cranial Sacral Therapy, Chiropractic

The first time I had cranial sacral therapy, I didn't feel anything, and it was so gentle I thought nothing could have happened. I went home, and later that evening, I felt very tired, went to bed and didn't get up for a week. Something had sure happened.

Over the week, though, I noticed positive changes in how I felt and when I got up, I realised that I felt stronger. In subsequent treatments, this abreaction was less severe until it didn't happen at all, and I just benefitted.

Movement therapies

Yoga, Tai Chi, Qi Gong, Biodynamic Psychotherapy, Feldenkrais

All these are usually very gentle forms of exercise and involve movement, breathing and meditation. I have done them all, and it's really a question of what you prefer. It's also worth mentioning that if something doesn't seem to be helping after two weeks, it probably won't after three, so it's time to try something else. Maybe later, it will help, so don't discount it altogether.

If you have ME/CFS, you probably have become restricted in your movements. The mere tension of "trying to hold yourself together" will also restrict your movement.

The muscle tension that arises when there is trauma in the body can be like armouring. Movement can involve emotional release.

I am at a yoga class, putting a bit of extra pressure on my arm to increase the range of my shoulder. Suddenly a memory comes up where my brother is forcing my arm up to my back (half nelson), and I start to cry as the tension releases. This lasts for only a few seconds, and then I feel relief and peace. I take a deep breath, and my shoulder gains some more movement.

Apart from the benefits of getting us gently moving, the movements of these modalities in themselves can help to balance our autonomic nervous system, help us learn to breathe correctly and help to "bring us home." By that, I mean to centre us, ground us and increase body awareness.

Tai chi has additional benefits, as the hands frequently cross over the midline of the body, helping to bring the two sides of our brain to work together. It is also very good for improving balance—and memory, as remembering the sequence can take some doing!

Qi Gong is a series of discreet exercises aimed at getting the body to move. It also involves breath, movement and balance.

Feldenkrais

A gentle way of re-establishing contact with the body, developed by Moshe Feldenkrais, involves very gentle exercises, just very small movements often done lying down.

Biodynamic Psychotherapy

I came across some books by Alexander Lowen—*Language of the Body*, *Fear of Life* and *Bioenergetics*—all about the way the body stores trauma. And then, I found Biodynamic Psychotherapy.

Biodynamic Psychotherapy does what it says. It uses many techniques to access trauma and release the resulting developed muscular armouring through the body and the mind.

Another similar therapy is Somatic Experiencing by Peter Levine.

I did a weekend workshop on Biodynamic Psycho-therapy, and it was the first time someone allowed me to "complete" a trauma. By that, I mean that I explained what I wanted to happen instead of what had happened by working through the memory of when I had my first panic attack. Then, by those present gently holding me and supporting me, I went through the event in a more supportive way.

The memory is: I am feeling seriously unwell. I think I am dying. My heart is racing, and I'm feeling sick and dizzy. I keep asking my colleague to take my pulse, but she refuses.

During the biodynamic workshop, I told the facilitator that I wanted my colleague to take my pulse. We go through the event, and when I ask the facilitator to take my pulse, she does, and I feel calmed and reassured by her presence and acceptance of my anxiety. My body relaxes.

I realised that my pulse rate at the workshop was not actually racing. Nevertheless, it helped to have my needs met, even if it was years after the event. I suppose, in modern parlance, I had closure.

Another interesting thing that I heard at this workshop was that, according to another bio-dynamic therapist, all the clients she had seen with ME/CFS had, at some time, damaged their tail bones or fallen heavily on their coccyx.

On searching the internet, I discovered that this is not an unknown phenomenon and that chiropractors do treat patients for fatigue associated with coccygeal injuries.

One day when I was 18, I was on horseback, learning to canter, when the horse veered suddenly to the right. I didn't and fell heavily on my bottom, fracturing a bone in my lumbar spine.

If you have had such a fall, then cranial-sacral or chiropractic treatment may help.

May you be free from fear

Chapter 12: Learning to Body Scan

Body Scanning is a learned skill and one that I think is well worth putting in the time to acquire. I have learned that my aches, pains, and many other sensations are stored memories and blocked emotions. As emotions seem to be energy in motion, we stop them and create aches, pains, and dis-ease by not allowing ourselves to feel the emotion. Body scanning has enabled me to discover and release these memories to continue my recovery.

It's often difficult to feel these feelings, especially if we were so overwhelmed by them in the first place that we repressed them. So, take baby steps—or what I refer to as nibbles—and then leave it alone for a bit.

Some emotions feel more unpleasant than others. I got used to allowing fear to arise, be felt and accepted, but I appreciate that fear can be completely overwhelming for some. Again, I remind you that you had felt this fear before and *survived*.

For me, shame was particularly toxic to experience. I felt dirty, debased, disgraced, and contaminated, and I was ashamed of being shameful, adding to the problem and increasing the tendency to block the emotion.

Another difficult emotion for me was anger. In fact, I didn't even recognise it for years as it was forbidden for me to be angry in my family—as for aggression, forget it! But both of these emotions are natural and part of the human personality. Suppressing them leads to problems, so they need to be expressed safely and appropriately.

I don't want to feel shame, and if the incident happened many years ago, I am not that shamed person now. I need to feel that shame and allow that younger me to grow up knowing that she is loveable despite these feelings.

Feelings and emotions also come and go, but we remain. The significance of this statement is that we are not our feelings or emotions even if we have temporarily identified ourselves with them.

Some people suggest working with the raw energy, and others suggest naming it. I do both; sometimes, one way works and sometimes the other.

Sometimes just working with a memory and not necessarily identifying the emotions works using tools such as the Emotional Freedom Technique or Havening.

Any emotion is defined as a continuum from one extreme to another, e.g., fear to love. They both arise simultaneously, but the other end is not known or experienced by focusing on one end. Having used The Journey many times on myself and with others, I know that there is always freedom and positive feelings at the other end. Being afraid to feel the fear sadly blocks us from love.

For example, a continuum might be:

Terror→anxiety→anger→emptiness→peacefulness→happiness→freedom→love

Or

Anger→rage→hate→contempt→hurt→sadness→peacefulness→love

"....in order not to fall ill, we must learn how to love..."
– Sigmund Freud

Or maybe it can also be said that we must learn how to love in order to recover.

Allowing the terror to be dissolved into love frees us from its grip, and we are healed, bit by bit. It's perfectly possible to do an internal body scan using your mind to discover the cause of the pain or symptom. We know where we are hurting, but not what that hurt might be. It's also possible to do an external body scan. But what are you looking for?

Simply put, areas that attract your attention. You may find that there is a feeling, a sensation, a hesitation as you scan that area, or an inner knowing that this area is somehow different, not at ease, wants to "tell" you something.

I lie down where I won't be disturbed and just try to relax. I observe my breathing. I breathe as evenly and rhythmically as possible. Starting from my toes or the top of my head, I take my awareness slowly through the inside of my body. Are there any areas that are tense or painful? Or

there may be warmth or cold, anything that is a bit different that catches and holds my attention.

I have a headache; I welcome it and tell it that I am listening. What does it want to say?

What am I feeling? There is pain. I breathe into the pain. Is it sharp or dull? It's dull and throbbing; I breathe and welcome that too. There is tightness, and I breathe into that.

If there was an emotion here, what would that be? Strangely, if I wait, I will be able to name an emotion.

Having named the emotion, I ask myself, when have I felt like this before? What is the core memory? Usually, I would get a little vignette of the scene. Seeing it from the maturity of my current age, I become aware that I don't need to be afraid anymore.

I developed this process following my hypnotherapy sessions with Wendy, and over time, I was able to do it wherever I was, whenever I needed it, rather than requiring a time out.

Emotions are, after all, a collection of sensations. If I asked you to be happy, you would know what to do, and then you could describe your feelings. Conversely, if I ask you what you are feeling, you could describe the sensations.

In this way, I learned about the traumas that were stored in my body, such as the belief that I need to please everybody. Simply knowing that eases the pressure and stress, I place on myself.

If I separate the feelings out and gently breathe into them, the emotion usually ceases to be overwhelming, and I can allow it to release and move. Over time and with practice, I have found all feelings can be accepted.

This scanning practice can be done daily or even immediately when something arises (if it's appropriate to stop and dialogue with it).

This is a hybrid method from several therapies, mainly from my hypnotherapy sessions with Wendy, but also from *The Journey*, Neuro-Linguistic Programming, Eckart Tolle's *The Power of Now*, etc.

Not only do we need to work with the emotion, but if there is a conflict in us, this needs to be resolved as well. For example, the conflict between being angry and the desire to be a "good" girl or boy. The conflict between being afraid and "big" girls or boys don't cry.

I was surprised how often the issues that were stored in my body were quite minor to me as an adult but were obviously traumatic to me as a little girl. Simply seeing them from my perspective now is enough to integrate and move on.

However, some emotions, some memories, are so severe that expert help is needed to face them. But remaining afraid to feel them means you cannot be released from their thrall.

As we release the hold these memories have on us, our bodies relax and become easeful. The more we do, the better they feel. The more pain and fear we release, the more love we can experience—and it's definitely a felt experience. And as I said earlier, "it's never too late to have a happy childhood," it's also never too late to have a comfortable body." Over time, it is possible to send this love that you are now discovering around your body to any part that you feel needs it.

Generate a feeling of love or gratitude right now by thinking of something that you love; maybe something in nature, a puppy or kitten, a friend, chocolate, anything that makes you feel warm, softer, and safer. Focus on that feeling. Where in your body do you feel it? Allow it to grow and expand to fill yourself up with these feelings. When you are overflowing with them, send them out into the world.

Establishing a gratitude practice will help with this. Start by thinking of three things you are grateful for, maybe the sun on your face, water (water is the most amazing stuff), that there is hope that you will recover. As you get better at this, enlarge your list to include three things about yourself that you appreciate.

Start and end the day with this.

May you be happy

Resources

The Journey by Brandon Bays

Bio-energetics by Dr Sue Morter

EFT

Havening

Chapter 13: The Problem with P.E.T.

Progressive or graduated exercise therapy is a system whereby the intensity of an exercise is increased gradually and was, at one time, advocated for people with ME/CFS, and many of you with ME/CFS will have been encouraged to do "a little more every day" only to discover that you can't.

As a physiotherapist, I was taught that this was the way to increase strength that the muscles would respond by getting stronger. If you could walk 20 yards one day, you should try and walk 20 + yards the next, and it always confused me when I was ill to find that one day I could walk, say, for 30 minutes and the next day I may not even be able to get out of bed.

Then there is "the line" over which you dare not cross! Even one step over it would put me in bed for 24-48 hours or more. What was going on?

I also had a problem with reading, in that just reading a few sentences, I would start to feel tired and ill.

What about watching television or any moving spectacle? Always used to make me feel very ill quite quickly, rather akin to seasickness.

Another of my symptoms was difficulty in changing focus rapidly. I would have to take my vision slowly across the floor to the new object I wanted to see, so I decided to try and do some eye exercises. I was scanning an eye chart up and down and suddenly knew that if I continued, I would trigger a panic attack.

It was as if my body had a mind of its own, and no matter how I tried to exercise or get stronger, it wouldn't let me.

What was going on?

The issue here, with the exercise of either the body or the eyes, is to do with your visual and vestibular apparatuses, involving the vestibular-ocular reflex.

Your vestibular apparatus or system is, in most mammals, the sensory system that contributes most to the sense of balance and spatial orientation (from Wikipedia). If it's off, you feel off.

There are many neuronal connections between your amygdala—the part of your brain that scans for danger—and the vestibular apparatus. This results in a close relationship between anxiety and balance disorders. Being stressed will disturb your balance, and if your balance is off, you need to work hard to maintain it. As you will know, people with ME/CFS can't stand for long.

I am at a wedding ceremony, and we are about to sing a hymn. I know that I can either stand or sing, but I do not have the energy to do both.

Scanning across the page when reading has a similar effect. This time, your head may be still, but your eyes are moving, sending signals to your vestibular apparatus, and, as written above, if it's off, you will feel off. It is the same as a moving horizon on a boat or any means of travel. Travel generally in any shape or form causes the horizon to move, triggering travel sickness in the susceptible—and the more sensitive you are, the more quickly it will happen. You are feeling "seasick" because you are hypersensitive now. Even though you are not moving, it's just your eyes that are moving.

It was also why I couldn't play tennis without having a panic attack or even run upstairs anymore. Why I couldn't read or watch any moving image without feeling anxious or nauseous. It was also why when I did feel those things that by looking at solid vertical lines it led to a reduction in anxiety and nausea. I had stabilized my horizon.

You need to make your brain happy again by resetting your vestibular apparatus. Ask yourself: is there an emotional issue residing in this system?

One day, I was trying, yet again, to ignore my illness by playing tennis. After a few games, I had to stop, I was feeling extremely anxious, and my heart was racing. I left the others to it and went to try and settle down.

I was pacing up and down, trying not to feel my beating heart. Just feeling it was fuelling my anxiety. Suddenly I had this insight "this is not killing me." The tachycardia vanished along with panic. It was so completely dramatic that I was astonished. I couldn't believe it.

What the "this" was, I have no idea, and I don't need to know. I also don't know where these insights, these "aha" moments come from, but most of us get them. They just seem to arise spontaneously. Maybe I suddenly understood that my heart could beat this quickly, and I wasn't going to die. Maybe it was that I was no longer moving my head and eyes a lot so everything could settle down, but it not only cured this episode, it has also been very long-lasting as I have only had one more attack since this, and this was 30 years ago.

During my recovery, I went to several personal trainers to help me with my goal of getting fitter. I would tell them my story, and they would nod and tell me they understood. Then I would have to go through their assessment and "just try one more," I was asked. Without fail, I would be ill four to six hours later (and why this delay? I don't know).

That is until I came across Graham at Simplicity Fitness. I told him my story, and he said, "Yes, I understand, and when your body tells you to stop—STOP."

The first exercises I ever did with Graham were to re-educate my vestibular apparatus. He asks me to hold my head still and follow a pointer with my eyes as he moves it from side to side and then up and down. If all was well, he would then move it around in a big circle.

Next, I would hold my eyes still and move my head from side to side and then up and down, etc.

If or as soon as I felt any discomfort, I would stop, look at a solid edge until the feeling passed, and then start again.

As soon as I felt any brain fog, I would know to stop and rest.

Slowly, slowly this problem was resolved, and I am rarely bothered by it now.

And it worked. Not only have I got a lot more strength and fitness back, but I am also more flexible. Because Graham has worked on retraining my vestibular apparatus as well as my overall strength and fitness, my body has been able to get out of hyper-vigilance and arousal into a relaxed state so I can move more. I have done yoga etc., for years, but because Graham helps me decommission flight or fight, I have access to more movement than any other method I've tried. And when I want to stop, I say so, and I stop. This also means I can trust him to care for me, and as he has said, "a happy mind for a happy body."

When I started to work with Graham, he never told me how many repetitions to perform. As he said, you know what you are feeling better than I do. Sometimes I did seven or ten, and other times, maybe only one. If the exercise involved lots of head movements, such as squats, then the number would probably be few.

Always feeling better after each session with no negative after-effects, I have made huge progress.

I do not understand the full picture of what happens and why we can feel so ill after exercise, but this is what I think may be happening.

Our bodies are stressed, they have been stressed for a long time, and we get ill. Then we rest a lot and feel a little better until we go and do something a little more. If we're very weak, it may simply be getting up, reading a book, watching TV, talking—anything that stimulates an exhausted nervous system and requires energy. But all our energy had been used up suppressing our emotions, which are now spilling forth. As they're negative emotions "attached" to the original trauma, we feel anxious or ill, and because we have forgotten the connection to the original trauma, they seem to come from nowhere.

As there is a big connection in the brain between our amygdala, which controls emotional responses (primarily fear), and the vestibular apparatus, hence balancing and recalibrating this apparatus is enormously beneficial to emotional regulation. Rebalancing calms the mind.

Several tests can show whether the vestibular apparatus needs help:

- Stand with your feet together, arms straight out in front, hands together.

- Turn your whole upper body and arms to the left, then to the right, and see how restricted your movements are.

- Stand with one foot in front of the other, toes of the back foot touching the heel of the front foot.

- Raise your arms in front of you.

- Close your eyes.

- Swap feet around and repeat.

(Above exercises developed by Dr. Eric Cobb and adapted by Graham Webber)

How unsteady are you? Is one way more unsteady than the other?

Make sure you're in a safe spot and can't hurt yourself.

Finding Pleasure

Simply doing something that gives you pleasure will cause your body to release feel-good hormones. For example, dopamine acts as a "reward" hormone, and endorphins will help relieve pain—something you really need if you suffer from ME/CFS. It can be just listening to good music, music that changes your mood, watching "happy" programmes, sitting in nature, and so on.

Somatic Experiencing, Body Stress Release

Somatic Experiencing was developed by Peter Levine as he resolved his own traumatic experiences.

A treatment that involves releasing the trauma from the body, it can be done in stages, called "pendulation," by Dr. Levine, or what I like to call "nibbles." When you've experienced a bit, and the feelings threaten to be overwhelming, you can withdraw to a safe psychic space that you have established beforehand, such as a perfect coral island, a green garden, or a woodland glade.

As the body releases the stored trauma, it's common to experience shaking. Although this is very safe and natural, in our "civilized" society, we tend to interpret the shaking as the issue, therefore adding to our trauma.

Watch any mammal after a frightening occurrence—it will shake itself free of the emotions. Natural history programs frequently show an antelope or other prey animal escaping from a predator, and minutes later, it is eating peacefully. It remains alert for danger but not neurotically so, stuck in fight-or-flight. However, humans tend to suppress this natural event and not release the trauma. We remain hypervigilant, not simply calmly vigilant.

EMDR, Brainspotting

EMDR stands for Eye Movement Desensitization and Reprocessing Technique and involves the client being gently reconnected to the thoughts, emotions, and sensations associated with the trauma. The patient then allows the natural healing power of the brain to recalibrate and adopt adaptive solutions. It's also part of the Havening technique, and it has certainly helped me.

I have only read about Brainspotting, as the closest practicing therapist was too far away for me to travel to regularly, but it works on a similar principle to EMDR: that the practice of moving the eyes can find stored memories which can then be worked with.

All these—and many other approaches that require one to be very focused on the movements—help us to "get back into our bodies." Even just walking can reacquaint you with your body if you do it mindfully. Notice how quickly or slowly you are walking, the length of your stride, the feel of the ground beneath your feet, your breathing, how your surroundings affect you, the feeling of the air on your skin, and so on.

May you be at peace

Resources

Exercises to recalibrate the vestibular apparatus. See YouTube

See also;

Dr. Eric Cobb

Applied Movement Neurology (AMN)

EMDR – www.psycom.net

Brainspotting by David Grand Ph.D.

Chapter 14: Meditation

Not long ago, meditation was considered somewhat fringe, but now, after much research, it's a mainstream practice that benefits most people. But if you have ME/CFS, the first question is, "how will it help me?"

Long-term meditators are about six years younger than non-meditators, but if you're suffering from ME/CFS, would you want to live another six years? Years of research have demonstrated that after a few meditation sessions, our biomarkers (blood pressure, sugar balance, and so on) are improved. So, let's get well!

I frequently hear people who give up on meditation say that they can't stop their thoughts, whatever they did. You probably won't either, because that's what brains and minds do, they think. The point of meditation is to observe our minds, distance ourselves from our thoughts, and challenge them and the habitual reactions that are triggered by both inside and outside events—including the things we do, the people we meet, the places we go and our thoughts. The point is to become aware that we are not our minds but the observer of our minds, bodies, thoughts, emotions, and feelings. All these things come and go, but we remain—so we cannot be these things. By observing our feelings and thoughts, we can become free of their influence, free to allow the energy to flow and to heal.

I found that life mirrored back exactly what I needed to learn about myself. In other words, I was increasing my awareness, and that brought healing.

Meditation will also allow you to still your mind so that you can become aware of all the emotions that you don't want to feel. This is not a threat and a reason not to meditate!

As we block our uncomfortable emotions, they become stored in our bodies. They don't go away, and we may adopt negative and self-destructive behaviours, including taking legal and illegal drugs, eating too much or too little, too much or too little sexing, over-and under-exercising, and so on in an effort to continue to block the emotions.

Meditation can help us allow whatever arises to be OK and accept it all without judgment or comment. To feel into it, gently but with persistence. To observe it and to let go of our identification with it. To move from a sense of "this is who I am" to "this is just a sensation arising in my body. I am not it."

When I started meditating, I found it incredibly difficult. My whole body wanted to get up and move. I could feel my right foot pressing hard into the floor, urging me to get up and go. So, I found a different way: I discovered music with binaural beats.

Binaural beat tapes send a slightly different tone to each ear, usually through headphones. The brain translates this into one tone, and it is believed that this can entrain the brain to different and more relaxed states. There is some debate about how it works, but I found the process beneficial. To paraphrase a UK advertising slogan, "binaural beats reach the parts that other methods don't."

By listening to these types of tapes, I was, in effect, being meditated. My brainwaves were being altered so that many of the repressed emotions were brought into my awareness. Often, especially at the beginning, this was an uncomfortable process, and my symptoms were briefly exacerbated. But over time, as I allowed the memories and associated feelings to emerge, I recovered and healed.

Frequently, what was felt in the body as severe discomfort, was of no major import to the adult me. Alarming and frightening for me as a four- or five-year-old, but easily dealt with as an adult.

"We can't solve problems by using the same kind of thinking we used when we created them." – Albert Einstein

By bringing adult awareness to the issues of our past histories—our inner child, the younger me, the younger you—we can solve our stored problems. We integrate and release. We heal.

I frequently thought that it was a cosmic joke that, although we don't want to feel these unpleasant feelings (and they can be seriously unpleasant), we do anyway because they are our symptoms. The symptoms may be in the form of pains, illnesses, or behaviours.

Another thought I have is that our illnesses and symptoms are akin to what Jung called the shadow. This unconscious part of us contains all that we don't know, are unaware of, and don't like about ourselves. But we also have a "golden shadow," which is equally unknown but contains the good bits—it's good to know these too.

"The most terrifying thing is to accept oneself completely." - Carl Jung.

"This thing of darkness, I acknowledge mine." – William Shakespeare

"Illness comes to heal us" – The Healing Power of Illness, Rüdiger Dahlke & Thorwald Dethlefsen

When we become aware of the feeling and are unafraid to feel it, not only are we free, but we also experience a curious sensation, a mixture of joy, love, and bliss. That is my day-to-day experience of life, so I have moved from feeling angry and tired, or other negative emotions, to a profound sense of fundamental wellbeing. That is why I know this way works.

There are many different types of meditation and if one doesn't suit, try another and if it stops working, try another.

May you be free from fear

Resources

Binaural Beat and Brainwave Entrainment

Numerous companies now make binaural and even trinaural (three tones) meditation tracks.

As small children, our brains mainly produce delta waves, so by entraining our brains to that same state, we have access to those childhood memories. As adults, we spend the most time in beta states unless we meditate, daydream, or sleep.

Holosync – www.centerpointe.com

iAwake Technologies – www.iawaketechnologies.com

Biofeedback devices that can be used to deepen your meditation practice:

Muse Headband

HeartMath's Inner Balance

Breathworks

Simply observing your own breath

HeartMath

Omnibreath

Mindfulness

Insight meditation (basically self-inquiry)

Mantra - any brief sentence or word that is repeated, e.g., love, your name, om

Chanting

Body scanning

"What is stopping the love from flowing?"

Walking, especially in woodland/forests

Simply sit with your back to a tree.

Chapter 15: A Few More Thoughts

Altruism

There are measurable effects on an individual from doing something for others; it seems that both you and the other person benefit. Maybe you are even more so than the person you're being altruistic toward.

I am seriously tired. I cannot stand for more than a few minutes. On most days, I can only walk very slowly for short distances when a friend of mine, involved in Riding for the Disabled, asks me to come along and help. I look at her in astonishment as she knows I am ill. "Oh, we don't want you to do anything. We just want your advice as a physiotherapist on how best to handle the children."

I went along, sat on the mounting block for an hour, returned home, and went to bed.

The next week I went along again, and after the session, the person leading the group approached me and started chatting. She was my introduction to an alternative way of understanding illness and disease and healing methods and, ultimately, my recovery.

Would this have happened anyway, without my willingness to help others while sick—and how can I know? But ask Lynne McTaggart. She doesn't know for sure either, but she has seen many examples of this in action. She has written a book about it called The Power of Eight, and it's well worth a read.

Do you even need to leave your home? No, you can join a healing intention group online, and even if it doesn't help you (although I suspect it will), it gives you something worthwhile to do, stopping the self-absorption that so frequently and quite naturally comes with ME/CFS or any illness.

Covid-19

I succumbed to Covid-19 right at the beginning of the lockdown in the UK and was very unwell with it. I was very surprised to get it. I suppose, like many people, I thought I was immune to everything, but no. And though I was quite seriously ill, I was lucky, as I did get through it.

Having got over the worse bit of it, fortunately, I was able to stay out of the hospital, but I took a few weeks to recover and was left with nausea, heart rhythm irregularities, and fatigue.

As I have come to think that most things have an emotional component, I started to wonder why I wasn't recovering and why I had my particular set of symptoms, along with what these symptoms were telling me.

It seemed to me that the virus had put my body on high alert, that I was using energy to recover, which had been used to suppress symptoms. Now they were here—big time.

I talked to a Lifestyle Prescriptions expert about my nausea and retching, which is often an inner ear problem leading to issues with balance. She said that these problems were associated with a fear of falling, being out of control, and/or balance, and I immediately had an "aha" moment. This was related to my feelings relating to horse riding and falling off horses.

I had always wanted to learn to ride horses as a little girl, but I was always afraid to "take the brakes off" when riding. However, I persevered—and then kept falling off the horse.

I had an accident when I was 18 and landed on my tail and another accident at 35 where I landed on my head. I also have had two experiences where I felt completely out of control.

In the first incident, I was riding through a small village when a bulldozer came around the corner. At the sight of this, the horse span around but luckily didn't bolt, as I think I would have been killed.

In the second one, I was out riding in a group, and the horse just took off, galloping across a field towards a gate. Was it going to jump over it? It was a small horse and a big gate, so fortunately for me, it stopped before the gate.

I decided to give up riding!

With that insight, my issues with nausea and retching resolved over the next 24-48 hours—but I was still left with the unpleasant irregular heartbeats.

I'd had these ever since I was 25 or so—not badly, and when I was checked out with all the usual tests, my heart was completely normal and healthy. However, when I became ill with ME/CFS, tachycardia was an issue. So, rhythm disturbances were not new to me.

I meditated on this issue for days; what was I feeling, what was my heart telling me, what was disturbing my peace and rhythm? What emotions were disturbing to me? What feelings didn't I want to feel? Suddenly I remembered an incident that took place when I was 17 and felt the intense anger that I had suppressed.

This memory was another part of the incident in the woods when I was being followed (see chapter 7). After the incident, I was overwhelmed with rage that my so-called friends had treated me like this and angry at myself for not confronting them about it. There was also rage at me over how I always suppressed my feelings to avoid challenging and confrontational situations.

Again, with this insight, the palpitations diminished and no longer troubled me. I carried this anger in my heart for over 50 years, and I didn't know it.

Following this insight, my energy is returning, and I have now turned the corner on my recovery. So even a virus has something to tell us, something to teach us from an inner perspective.

Also, I didn't suffer the severe lung symptoms associated with Covid-19, so perhaps lung issues (which, according to meta-health and Lifestyle Prescriptions, are related to territorial fear or fright) are not my issues.

Kundalini and Spiritual Emergencies

I am reluctant to write on this topic as there are whole books written about it, and what I can say here will be very cursory. However, I think it is important to mention it because, from my reading, ME/CFS could be mistaken for an uncontrolled and spontaneous arising of the Kundalini energy in someone unprepared.

What is Kundalini? According to Hindu tradition, the body's life force lies coiled like a snake at the base of the spine. As it arises, it purifies the body/mind and causes buried emotions and memories to be brought to the surface to be integrated. If this process is not understood, the whole affair can be alarming, if not downright terrifying. Suddenly you are experiencing all these weird feelings, and many of them are identical to the symptoms reported in ME/CFS. Though if you prepare the way properly, this energy rises unhindered, bringing states of bliss.

The kundalini energy wants to shake the blocked emotions free; your body might spontaneously move and twitch to do this. These movements are often snake-like or sinuous. It is a healing, enlightening process but not without some challenges for the unprepared.

This kundalini process appears to be self-directed, but you can work with it or against it. By resisting your feelings and trying to block the emotions, you are working against them. Many of the body/mind therapies available today will help the energy blocks release, assisting the process and helping you feel better. Every time you release a blockage, you become more whole, more integrated, as the parts you had cut off become constructive parts of you. In the end, no emotion is seen as bad or wrong. Does that mean you vent anger, aggression, hatred, etc., at anyone? No, you learn to use these energies safely, transform your life, and maybe later transform the lives of others where you see injustice, mistreatment, or deprivation.

We have tended to separate the mind and the body in both medicine and spiritual practices in the West. But now is the time to unite and integrate them. The body is not to be mistreated to attain spiritual growth. I have said elsewhere that I used my body to heal my mind and my mind to heal my body. My body's symptoms show that I still have mental, emotional, and spiritual work to do, and this energy is trying to cleanse and heal me. It is an ongoing process.

As I said above, raising one's kundalini appears to be a self-directed process in that one thing leads to or exposes another. But I would recommend being under the guidance of an experienced practitioner. In hindsight, I am amazed at how I was led by the universe from book to person to therapy in a way that would have been impossible for me to work out myself. After all, what did I know? I'd not even heard of kundalini at the time I was affected. I usually got the information just before I needed it!

I also had to trust. Once I accepted that a spontaneous kundalini arising had probably occurred, I started to trust the process and that all would ultimately be well. That did not mean it was an easy path. I still had to feel the feelings and integrate and forgive. I still had to do the work.

Diet & Supplements

I know very little about diet and supplements because it wasn't the focus of my approach to healing. I did try the "caveman diet" for a while and swapped one load of symptoms for another.

However, there was a major benefit in cutting out sugar as my blood sugar became much more balanced.

I would advise good, healthy, preferably chemical-free food, and as little processed as possible, but that is common sense.

I know that many people with chronic fatigue have food intolerance issues, and I did too, but as I've recovered, they have gone.

Regarding supplements, I recommend a good probiotic to enhance your gut health. Good gut health is now known to be very important for our overall health and wellbeing. A co-enzyme Q10 supplement supports our energy production systems: I will refer you to Dr. Sarah Myhill's book, Chronic Fatigue Syndrome and Myalgic Encephalomyelitis, for more thorough information than I can give you on supplements. And "The China Study" by T. Colin Campbell and his son Thomas for good dietary suggestions.

Doing Something That Pleases You

It doesn't matter what you do, but doing something that pleases you creates feel-good hormones in your body—and feeling good is in seriously short supply when you have ME/CFS.

Doing this could be simply listening to music, watching funny films (but don't overdo them as laughing changes your breathing), painting, playing with a pet, walking, or sitting in nature.

May you be happy

Resources

Power of Eight Groups - Lynne McTaggart www.lynnemctaggart.com

Add Heart - info@weaddheart.com

Meditation

HeartMath

Breathwork

Havening Technique

EFT

Massage

Yoga

Tai Chi

Qi Gong

Lifestyle Prescriptions

For help with kundalini - bonniegreenwell.com

Spiritual Emergency Network

Chapter 16: And Finally

Where has all this work led me? Certainly, it has led me to heal myself and gain a profoundly deep sense of well-being. Having integrated my traumas, having forgiven the "perpetrators," having released my stored memories, I am left with feeling a delightful mixture of love, joy, and happiness. My heart feels open, my body, despite its 70+ years, is pain-free, and I welcome life's experiences. I no longer shy away, armour myself, or feel a need to defend myself.

My recovery has taken me from a debilitating illness, suicidal thoughts, and hopelessness to joy and happiness. It has surely been a gift in disguise.

Sure, stuff happens, it always has, and it always will, but I can deal with it. I have learned to be resourceful, and I always will be because I have discovered our essential nature; being, awareness, and bliss. I am not only free from ME/CFS but free from me—or rather, the me I thought I was. I've lost the limited, inadequate, frightened me and become happy and free.

I hope that some of the ideas presented here will help you find your own way through. It's not an easy route, but it is worth it. The courage to face our demons, to move from pain and disease to a life of joy and peace, lives within us. We can change, we can heal, and we can grow. Our past is not our future.

In the beginning, I wanted to be rescued from what I knew not. Everything I did was an effort to escape my past by moving away from it, but that didn't work as I just came along too. When I stopped, turned, and faced my demons, I opened the path to change and heal. I hope you find your way, and I hope you find the support and assistance that you may need as you heal. We don't have to do this alone.

Congratulations to you for taking this first step by reading this book—it takes great courage to try a new way. I wish you the speediest of recoveries.

To New Beginnings:

May you be happy

May you be well

May you be free from fear

May you be at peace

And may you be filled with loving-kindness

DID3431578

L - #0341 - 251122 - C0 - 229/152/8 - PB - DID3431578